THE CHALLENGE OF
FAMILY THERAPY
A Dialogue for Child Psychiatric Educators

THE DOWNSTATE SERIES OF
RESEARCH IN PSYCHIATRY AND PSYCHOLOGY

A Continuation Order Plan is available for this series. A continuation order will bring delivery of each new volume immediately upon publication. Volumes are billed only upon actual shipment. For further information please contact the publisher.

THE CHALLENGE OF FAMILY THERAPY

A Dialogue for Child Psychiatric Educators

Edited by

Kalman Flomenhaft
and
Adolph E. Christ

Downstate Medical Center
Brooklyn, New York

PLENUM PRESS · NEW YORK AND LONDON

Library of Congress Cataloging in Publication Data

Main entry under title:

The Challenge of family therapy.

(The Downstate series of research in psychiatry and psychology; v. 3)
Proceedings of the Conference on Family Therapy in the Training of Child Psychiatrists,
sponsored by and held at the Department of Psychiatry, Downstate Medical Center, Brook-
lyn, New York, New York, December 8–9, 1978.
   Includes index.
   1. Family psychotherapy—Congresses. I. Flomenhaft, Kalman. II. Christ, Adolph. III. New
York (State). Downstate Medical Center, New York. Dept. of Psychiatry. IV. Series: Down-
state series of research in psychiatry and psychology; v. 3. [DNLM: 1. Family therapy—
Education—Congresses. 2. Child psychiatry—Education—Congresses. W1 DO945 v. 3/WM18
C437
RC488.5.C45   616.98′156   80-18943
ISBN 978-1-4684-3847-5   ISBN 978-1-4684-3845-1 (eBook)
DOI 10.1007/978-1-4684-3845-1

Proceedings of the Conference on Family Therapy in the Training of
Child Psychiatrists, sponsored by and held at the Department of Psychiatry,
Downstate Medical Center, Brooklyn, New York, December 8–9, 1978.

© 1980 Plenum Press, New York
Softcover reprint of the hardcover 1st edition 1980
A Division of Plenum Publishing Corporation
227 West 17th Street, New York, N.Y. 10011

FOREWORD

This volume on Family Therapy Training, edited by Kalman Flomenhaft, Ph.D. and Adolph E. Christ, M.D., is the outgrowth of a successful conference on Family Therapy in the Training of Child Psychiatrists sponsored by the Department of Psychiatry at the Downstate Medical Center on December 8 and 9, 1978. The attendance and enthusiastic participation at this conference reflected the growing interest on the part of psychiatrists and other mental health professionals in the theory, practice, and teaching of family therapy.

That the conference was held at all presupposed the value that psychiatric educators are attaching to the incorporation of family therapy teaching in the educational development of psychiatrists. While the conference was dedicated to family therapy training for child psychiatrists, this volume is broadened to include family therapy training for all psychiatrists and mental health professionals. The various chapters delineate the issues in the teaching of family therapy, both theoretical and practical. The richness of the chapters that follow grows out of the depth of practical experience of the various authors in developing family therapy training in established programs where resistance to new ideas as well as structural changes in curriculum are predictable. The nature of both the theoretical and practical aspects of such resistances is well described. The authors also emphasize what is required to launch a successful training program in child psychiatry, stressing the importance of attractive role models as teachers of family therapy.

Anyone interested in the education of psychiatrists as well as nonpsychiatric mental health professionals will find this volume extremely useful because of the large reservoir of experience from which it derives.

Eugene B. Feigelson, M.D.
Professor and Chairman
Department of Psychiatry
Downstate Medical Center
Brooklyn, New York

PREFACE

     This volume is derived from the symposium "Family Therapy in
the Training of Child Psychiatrists" which was held in December,
1978 at Downstate Medical Center. A number of leading psychiatric
educators and family therapists gathered together to acknowledge
the significance of family therapy in training child psychiatrists
and other mental health practitioners.

     For two days the participants, through a series of prepared
papers and dialogue with each other, shared their beliefs and
experiences. They grappled with significant theoretical and
practical issues of clinical training and practice. All the contributions were marked by an intellectual enthusiasm and commitment
to examine the variety and complexity of the issues. Points of
agreement and disagreement among the participants were honestly
acknowledged and considered.

     The symposium proceedings were recorded on audio-tape in their
entirety and edited for the purposes of this volume. The editors
are grateful to Mrs. Beverley DeSouza for her help with the hundreds
of details in arranging the symposium and preparing this volume.
Thanks are expressed to Mrs. Libby Cohen in organizing the symposium,
Mr. Martin Nathanson for the audio recording of the proceedings,
and to Mrs. Caroline Apolito and Mrs. Liela Berger in deciphering
the final manuscript.

     We deeply appreciate the support and encouragement provided
by our families throughout the entire process of the symposium and
the editing of the proceedings.

     Finally, the editors are most grateful to the Elizabeth
Berliss-Saenger, M.D. Memorial Fund for sponsoring this symposium.

Kalman Flomenhaft, Ph.D.

Adolph E. Christ, M.D.

CONTENTS

INTRODUCTION: THE CHALLENGE OF FAMILY THERAPY

Kalman Flomenhaft, Ph.D.

Downstate Medical Center-Kings County Hospital

Brooklyn, New York 11203

The introduction of a new way of thinking about and treating psychiatric problems is fraught with difficulties and resistances. A profession becomes wedded to one approach, and the tendency is to stay with that one. For a member of a profession to consider and accept new ideas might undermine long-established and cherished beliefs and practices. These new ideas could represent a threat to what the individual has been doing all along. This is not very attractive to those who have devoted lifetimes to the acquisition of concepts and therapeutic techniques whose prior assumptions are now being questioned. As a psychiatrist colleague said, "Let's face it, I have too much at stake in this thing to change now. I have helped a lot of people over the years, so I must have been doing something right."

Therefore, it is not mere coincidence that new treatment approaches originate often from outside the more traditional professional institutions and from individuals not usually in leadership positions. These ideas are advanced and developed by younger members of the profession and from related disciplines in semi-professional and fringe settings.

BEGINNINGS OF FAMILY THERAPY

The beginnings of family therapy in the 1950's and early 1960's, understandably, occurred in settings like the Mental Research Institute of California and the Jewish Family and Children's Service of New York City. Neither was associated with major psychiatric training institutions. Though some of the early pioneers came from the principal mental health disciplines of psychiatry (Ackerman, 1958; Bowen, 1960; Jackson, 1959), psych-

1

ology (McGregor, 1964), and social work (Satir, 1964), major contributions were made by Gregory Bateson (1956) and Jay Haley (1963)
an anthropologist and communications specialist, respectively.

Interest in family therapy expanded greatly for a variety of
reasons. The previously mentioned settings offered a wide range
of family therapy training programs which attracted large numbers
of mental health professionals. Significant publications by the
above-mentioned pioneers, including the founding of the Journal
of Family Process in 1962, did much to advance family therapy.
In addition to their publications, they took to the road like
missionaries, conducting workshops and seminars in various locales
throughout the country. As teachers of family therapy, they
concluded that the best way to convince people of what they were
doing was to demonstrate the doing. Consequently, considerable
use was made of audio-visual technology including video tape, film,
and live demonstrations of actual family therapy interviews. This
contributed greatly towards promoting the family therapy movement.

During the late 60's, the novelty of seeing an entire family
together seemed to be over. Clearly, family therapy was developing into something more than a passing fad. The works of
S. Minuchin (1967) and Langsley (1968) demonstrated the application
of family therapy concepts and techniques in working with the
families of juvenile delinquents from urban ghettos and acutely
psychotic individuals. Both these reports had a strong research
component which validated the clinical effectiveness of family
therapy. Finally, the report issued by the Group for the Advancement of Psychiatry (1970) further legitimized the family therapy
approach.

The appeal of family therapy was heightened, too, because of
the social climate during the 60's. Those times were marked by
a high rate of divorce and family break-up, less interest in
traditional family values and the development of alternative
family and community life styles. By focusing on the family, the
importance of the family was maintained through some very difficult
times when family life was being besieged.

Increasing acceptance and legitimization of family therapy
led to its gradual introduction into service programs and training
curricula of major psychiatric centers. The early advocates and
adherents began to assume clinical and educational leadership
positions for the development of family therapy programs. Now
the next stage was being confronted. How to translate these ideas
into viable service and training programs? They faced a wide
range of organizational, administrative, clinical, and educational
challenges in attempting to work with and teach about families.
An organization's tradition, hierarchy, and procedures inter-

digitate critically with the treatment services and training
programs being conducted. With a dash of cynicism, Haley (1975)
suggested that these obstacles are so great that some psychiatric
centers should avoid offering family therapy. Undaunted by these
obstacles, however, the early advocates established family oriented
programs at major psychiatric centers throughout the country.

The 70's have been marked by a mushrooming of family therapy.
It is increasingly becoming a part of the training of all mental
health professionals. A body of knowledge and experience is
developing which deserves careful consideration. A symposium was
convened at the Downstate Medical Center Department of Psychiatry
in December, 1978, to bring together leading authorities, intimately involved in the development and conduct of family therapy
training, to examine the issues and experiences which relate to
this body of knowledge. Some of these areas are the structure
and content of family therapy theory and training, including a
typology of the various family therapy approaches; obstacles that
have been encountered in introducing family therapy in the clinical
programs and training curricula of mental health organizations
and how they have been resolved; how it is taught and the nature
of clinical supervision; as well as descriptions of how the teaching of family therapy is or is not integrated with other areas of
training.

These authorities were invited to prepare papers relating
to the above issues in advance of the symposium. Each paper was
critiqued by another symposium participant. This volume is a
compilation of the papers and their critique as well as their
discussion by the symposium participants and the registrants.

Though the major focus is on family therapy training for
child psychiatrists, the content has relevance for training of
all the psychiatric disciplines. This document will be of
interest to practitioners, teachers, and supervisors of family
therapy training programs for social workers, psychologists,
nurses, and other mental health disciplines.

FAMILY THERAPY AND CHILD PSYCHIATRY

As with all the other mental health disciplines, child
psychiatry is now seriously considering the significance and
implications of family theory and therapy. No longer is it
acceptable and sufficient to declare that the child lives and
functions in a social context of parents, siblings, families,
peers, neighborhood, community, and schools. No longer is it
acceptable merely to say that these are factors for consideration.
Family theory compels us to go beyond the passivity of mere
consideration to the challenge of how can we integrate these

factors into our understanding and treatment of the child and
family. And as we move in this direction, let us be quite clear
that this is a major shift in thinking. This is a painful shift
for some, that becomes clear as we examine and question the
assumptions and perspectives that shape our thinking and practice.
We are creatures of habit and most comfortable with our usual
ways of conducting our business.

Clearly, though, the inherent soundness and reasonableness
of the family therapy position compels us to alter our views and
take on the challenge of these ideas. The question of the what
and why of family therapy is now being asked with greater deference
and certainly less vituperation than in the past. Times have
changed considerably since McDermot (1974) wrote "The Undeclared
War between Child and Family Therapy." The war is over, and
there is movement towards detente and more peaceful co-existence.

DOWNSTATE MEDICAL CENTER - CHILD PSYCHIATRY

As the host institution for the symposium, it is only
fitting to describe the past and current state of family therapy
within the Division of Child and Asolescent Psychiatry of Downstate Medical Center. Just because we are the host is no
indication that this is a paradise for family therapy, any more
or less free of the problems associated with the development and
conduct of family therapy to be found in any other setting.

At Downstate Medical Center, the history of family therapy
training goes back about 10 years to 1969. It then became an
integral part of the training curriculum with seminars on theory
and practice techniques, with opportunities for live and videotape supervision. During the first six years, there were
restricted criteria for the kinds of families considered appropriate for treatment; the families needed to be intact, and no
member of the family diagnosed as paranoid. The Division has
moved considerably from those times towards a more inclusive
view with a much wider range of families currently considered
appropriate for treatment.

As time has moved on, family therapy has moved well beyond
being only an interesting and exotic part of the training
curriculum. More of a family oriented approach has been integrated
into the service delivery system of our children's outpatient
clinic, and for the last several years, all initial evaluation
contacts are made with the entire family with a noticeable
increase in the number of families being seen as a unit. This is
a major shift and a sign of the increasing acceptance of more
family oriented services.

Currently, the curriculum for the child fellows contains didactic seminars in family therapy which includes discussion of the literature, observing live and video tape interviews of family therapy and, above all, opportunities for live and recorded supervision of the trainees' work with families. Medical students, residents in psychiatry, social work students, art therapy interns, psychology interns, and others are also offered family therapy seminars and practicums.

SYMPOSIUM ISSUES

During two very intense and wintry days in December, 1978, the symposium presenters shared their ideas and experiences as administrators, practitioners, teachers, supervisors of family therapy clinical and training programs. They systematically posed and analyzed the following vital clinical and training problems and issues, offering some solutions and directions for the future.

The trainee often has a difficult conceptual transition to make from an individual orientation to a systems family one. For some, it is a quantum leap. As one trainee said, "I am used to thinking and dealing with only one person. To talk with more than one person in a room is extremely difficult and anxiety provoking." It can be an overwhelming task for a beginner to relate to a family whose members may range in age from one day to 70 plus years, males and females, in a variety of roles, including son, daughter, mother, father, sibling, grandparents, etc.

The challenge is further heightened because of the nature of the patient population which often compels the trainee to go beyond the immediate family and to consider social, community, and environmental influences in a more ecological approach. A significant percentage of the patient population seen in our clinics are socially, educationally, and economically disadvantaged. Clearly, these families must be understood in their total context if, indeed, the therapeutic process is going to prove effective.

As a rule, family therapy requires more of a current here and now approach in observing, relating, and interacting to the family's sequences of verbal and nonverbal patterns of communication behavior. The significance of the present which is happening right in front of the trainee's eyes as a diagnostic and a treatment opporunity fails to be considered. By dint of his or her previous training, the trainee is much more comfortable dealing with the past, taking history, externalizing events and situations, and ignoring what is currently taking place within the life space of the family.

The age and life experiences of some of the trainees are highlighted as they confront families. Their own level of personal
and social development may limit the capacity to relate to
families. Some of them may be unmarried, and if married, have
no children, with many still in the throes of disengaging from
their own families of origin. This lack of life experience
handicaps some trainees to take therapeutic leadership roles with
families.

Moving from the more individual trainee concerns, the
symposium deals with the process of introducing family therapy
into organizations which had been predominantly individually
oriented. The administrative, staff, clinical, and training
considerations associated with the process are elucidated.
Several of the papers describe the various ways this process was
carried out and the results obtained. Finally, the major part of
the symposium outlines the goals of child psychiatry education and
the relationship to family therapy. The components of a number
of family therapy training programs including the content of the
didactic seminars and the nature of the supervisory process are
described. This varies with the orientation of the training
institution, depending whether the family approach is integrated
with other theoretical frameworks or is the singular orientation.
This struggle permeates the content of all the formal presentations
and dominates the stimulating and exciting panel discussion which
concludes the two-day symposium.

REFERENCES

Ackerman, N. W. Psychodynamics of Family Life: Diagnosis and
    Treatment in Family Relationships. New York:Basic Books,
    1958.
Bateson, G., Jackson, D. D., Haley, J. and Weakland, J. Towards
    a Theory of Schizophrenia. Behavioral Science, 1956, 1,
    251-264.
Bowen, M. A Family Concept of Schizophrenia. In: D. D. Jackson
    (Ed.), The Etiology of Schizophrenia. New York:Basic Books,
    1960.
Group for the Advancement of Psychiatry, Committee on the Family.
    The Field of Family Therapy. New York, 1970.
Haley, J. Strategies of Psychotherapy. New York:Grune and
    Stratton, 1963.
Haley, J. Why a Mental Health Clinic Should Avoid Family Therapy.
    Journal of Marriage and Family Counseling, 1975, 1, 3-13.
Jackson, D. D. Family Interaction, Family Homeostasis, and Some
    Implications for Conjoint Family Psychotherapy. In: I. J.
    Masserman (Ed.), Individual and Familiar Dynamics, New York:
    Grune and Stratton, 1959.
Langsley, D., and Kaplan, D. The Treatment of Families in Crisis.
    New York: Grune and Stratton, 1968.

McDermott, J. and Char, W. The Undeclared War Between Child and Family Therapy. Journal of American Academy of Child Psychiatry, 1974, 13, 422-436.

McGregor, R., Ritchie, A. M., Serrano, A. C., Schuster, F. P., McDonald, E. C. and Goolishan, H. A. Multiple Impact Therapy With Families, New York: McGraw-Hill, 1964.

Minuchin, S., Montalvo, B., Guerney, B. G., Rosman, B. L. and Shumer, F. Families of the Slums: An Exploration of Their Structure and Treatment, New York:Basic Books, 1967.

Satir, V. M. Conjoint Family Therapy: A Guide to Theory and Technique. Palo Alto: Science and Behavior Books, 1964.

TEACHING FAMILY THERAPY TO PSYCHIATRIC RESIDENTS AND CHILD

PSYCHIATRY FELLOWS: A DEPARTMENT CHAIRMAN'S POINT OF VIEW

Donald G. Langsley, M.D.

University of Cincinnati, College of Medicine

Cincinnati, Ohio

INTRODUCTION AND BASIC CONCEPTS

Ten years ago we might have debated whether family therapy should be part of the core training in adult psychiatry or child psychiatry. Today we discuss how to do it rather than whether to do it. Family therapy is now considered a required topic in the accreditation of both adult and child psychiatry. The skills related to family evaluation and treatment as well as knowledge about family psychology are no longer novelties. In a recent survey of 300 teachers of psychiatry as well as a random sample of 200 practitioners, 72% of the group felt that knowledge about basic concepts of family organization definitely should be included in the repertoire of the specialists in psychiatry and 28% felt that such knowledge should probably be included. In terms of clinical skills, the same group felt that a specialist in psychiatry should definitely be able to conduct a family interview (81%) and another 16% felt that this skill should probably be included. These attitudes about family therapy come from broad advances in the field and from wide clinical experience which has demonstrated the usefulness of family evaluation and family therapy to the psychiatrist. During the past quarter century, we have come to recognize that family psychology may be an organizing principle for teaching about normal and abnormal behavior of individual and groups. The family has come to be viewed as a psychological as well as a sociological unit. Not only does the family have a major influence on individual behavior, but it is seen as a basic resource and primary unit for intervention at a time of trouble. Family therapy is not just a special or different kind of treatment such as psychodynamic psychotherapy or transactional analysis; it is an approach meant to deal with basic causes of maladaptation. The family is not another social support system for which a substitute may be found in times of trouble. It is the basic unit of social psychology. Family therapy is not simply another approach to understanding the individual, but family theories may be conceived from dynamic and developmental points of view. The effort of the clinician should be to understand the family itself and not just its relationship to its individual components.

Family interviews provide a three dimensional demonstration of behavior since the family therapist can sit back and watch family interaction as it occurs. The one-to-one therapist gets a two dimensional report of something which occurred "out there" and sometimes is able to obtain corroboration from collateral interviews. Even these data are ignored by the psychiatrist who entertains the mystique of never seeing members of the family because it will interfere with one-to-one therapy. The psychology of family has made a number of contributions to psychiatry. It represents an opportunity to teach systems theory and to demonstrate systems concepts in action. Concepts of communication are a "natural" for approaching families rather than individuals. The field of family therapy has evolved a number of theoretical contributions which enhance the understanding of the family and which have developed a psychology of family theory. In addition, the clinical opportunity to see families presents the teacher with a situation in which to demonstrate concepts of homeostasis, complementarity, and even concepts of prevention when there is contact with the family over a long period of time. It should be recognized from the outset that family theory is meant to broaden an understanding of the individual as well as the family. It is not viewed as a substitute for individual psychology or a suggestion that only families (never individuals) should be the unit of clinical treatment.

CORE KNOWLEDGE IN UNDERSTANDING FAMILIES

The field of family classification is still one in which clinical description predominates. To date we have not developed a satisfactory approach to classifying and describing families. It will be easier to do research on the effectiveness of family therapy and the proper approaches to training in family therapy when we can manage family diagnosis more reliably. Actually, there is a body of knowledge which is developing and a discussion of teaching family therapy should take that into account. A psychodynamic approach to family interaction might include data on intimacy or power or boundaries. Cuber and Harroff (1966) have classified marital intimacy on a continuum which ranges from "conflict-habituated" to "vital" or even "total" of marriage.

They list "devitalized" or "passive-congenial" as stages between the two ends of the continuum, though these measures are predominantly descriptive and suggest alterations in family dynamics on the theme of power as a dynamic of interaction. In terms of intimacy, Lederer and Jackson (1968) have classified these dynamics in terms of symmetrical, complementary and parallel relationships. Symmetrical relationships assume equality and similarity of roles, whereas in complementary relationships, the differences are maximized. Parallel relationships occur where there is appropriate alteration between realistic symmetrical and complementary needs. A third dynamic approach focuses on boundaries. This issue describes who or what is part of the family relationship. When friends become as close as a spouse or a substitute for intimacy, one can see a boundary issue in the family. The "workaholic" has a family conflict which reflects a struggle between work and family. These dynamic approaches (power, intimacy, and boundaries) offer a body of theory which permits a psychodynamic understanding of the family to be tested.

A developmental point of view for the family is also gradually emerging. A psychodynamic classification of the family is predominantly cross-sectional, but families change over time and a developmental approach needs to be added to account for longitudinal change and crises. Berman and Leif (1975) have suggested a developmental approach to understanding marriage relationships which may be viewed as a model for extension to the whole family. The schema is one which defines tasks specific to a stage of the marriage and which outlines potential psychodynamic as well as developmental events for that time. This is one example of how developmental information can be organized so as to combine a useful approach to the understanding of the family.

In addition to core knowledge about the dynamic and developmental points of view, a great deal of research has been published on families which include a schizophrenic member. This topic was one of the earliest areas of interest and points to a number of reasons why a knowledge about families should be included in the core curriculum of the child psychiatrist and the adult psychiatrist. The fact that there is such a large body of data on families of schizophrenic patients, suggests the importance of family psychology to other psychiatric conditions. Other family studies have focused on the effectiveness of family therapy itself. In Gurman and Kniskern's (1978) review of the literature on this topic, they point to the fact that there are a number of completed and published studies which demonstrate the effectiveness of family therapy. They also highlight the need for more careful design and controls for comparison groups. Though the field is relatively young, it is comforting to note that some research has been done and that there is a body of knowledge which can be reviewed. These are the types of knowledge which should be part of the curriculum in teaching family therapy.

CORE SKILLS

     The issues around teaching family therapy must define the core
skills necessary to this field and must develop techniques for
teaching them. The basic skills might include: (1) the ability
to do a family diagnostic interview; (2) the ability to decide
when to see the family (or some subgroup of the family) or an
individual member or both; (3) the ability to do crisis intervention
and/or short-term treatment with the family; (4) the ability to do
family therapy for long-term problems. As with most clinical
disciplines, the didactic information (knowledge) generally
precedes actual experience, but must be integrated with it. For
adult psychiatry residents, one might propose a didactic course
on family theories to precede the clinical experience. This
didactic seminar is then followed by demonstrations of family
interviews. Afterwards the student is given opportunity to evaluate
families (diagnostic interviews) and to discuss them with a teacher-
supervisor. The next step in the sequence consists of supervised
experience in doing both short-term and long-term family therapy.
The general principle is to "watch one, do one, teach one" as the
student moves on to supervise others. For the child psychiatry
resident (fellow), the educational program is more complicated.
Some child fellows have had their adult psychiatry in the same
department as they will have their child training, while others
come from a different department. The preparation for family
diagnostic interviews and family therapy will differ according to
prior experience. It may be necessary to repeat the entire
sequence--at least briefly reviewing the didactic material
necessary to understand families since some trainees will not have
had it during adult psychiatry residency.

TEACHING TECHNIQUES

     Liddle and Halpin (1978) have recently reviewed the litera-
ture on teaching family therapy, and cite 105 publications touching
on this topic. The breadth of the field is suggested by the many
points of view about how to teach family therapy. To some the
task is accomplished by creating an atmosphere wherein family
therapists can grow by learning from experience. To others, a more
cognitively based approach is used to develop defined therapist
competencies in an organized fashion. Techniques have been
discussed which include:

     1. Block or integrated teaching. Should family therapy be
a sequence taught in all years of the program or should it be

concentrated in one block? Those who view family as an organizing
principle and as important as the individual "patient" favor a
sequence which is integrated throughout the total program.

2. Sequence and timing. As noted above, a favored approach
is to offer didactic seminars early in the training. This is
followed by family diagnosis (often demonstrated by videotapes)
and followed by supervised experience in family evaluation. Those
who use the block approach or who limit the time devoted to family
therapy are likely to stop here, while others go on to supervised
experience in brief and long-term family therapy. The block
approach generally offers a brief experience late in the residency
(sometimes as elective only) while the integrated teaching generally
begins early in the program and continues throughout it.

3. Didactic versus experiential. This issue concerns whether
didactic instruction is sufficient to make an effective family
therapist. Most teachers would agree that supervised clinical
experience is essential. Others feel that the therapist should
"experience" family (or marital) therapy as a patient and propose
that it be part of the training program. There is no agreement
on this issue, nor is there data to substantiate one position or
another. Some teachers approach this by using the classroom
situation to have each student construct a family genogram. Some
students are "turned off" by this approach and become very
defensive about looking at their own families; others find this
approach stimulating and useful. To date there is no way to
compare family therapy for the family therapist to personal psychotherapy for the individual therapist. In the latter case it is
presumed that therapy will help to deal with those personal
problems which inhibit one's effectiveness as an individual psychotherapist. There is no theoretical position about countertransference on a family basis or data about the connections between
trouble in one's own family and complications in doing family
therapy.

4. Who is qualified to teach? Family therapy is new enough
not to have become over-organized. Though there are groups of
family therapists who meet within other organizations, there is
no definitive professional group, nor is there a well-accepted
credentialing process. Family therapists come from diverse professional backgrounds. Some have acquired their skills and
experience in organized programs and others are self-taught.
Education takes place as part of a recognized university program
in some areas. In other regions, "family institutes" have arisen
outside of university programs in response to a lack of enthusiasm
for family therapy in the universities. The credentials to call
oneself a family therapist or a supervisor have not been established. Family therapists are self-defined and self-appointed.

5. <u>How does supervision work?</u> Supervision of clinical work
is considered the keystone in learning family therapy. The types
of supervision vary from the traditional technique of the supervisor listening to a report of a family session to closer involvement in the process of the therapy itself. Videotapes have
made it possible to conveniently demonstrate family therapy and
to watch and teach it. The use of "live supervision" has expanded
recently, and this varies all the way from the "supervisor" sitting
in the session as a "co-therapist" to direct observation by the
supervisor and commenting afterwards. The supervisor may even
intervene in the session as it is taking place by giving suggestions
over a private audio-communication channel or by interrupting the
session and coming into the room from behind a one-way screen.

PROBLEMS IN TEACHING FAMILY THERAPY

This review of family therapy teaching should also take note
of some of the problems. One of the major ones is that fact that
the senior faculty in any fellowship or residency program generally
do not do family therapy. Since the field is relatively new, this
skill is often demonstrated and advocated by junior faculty. The
senior faculty who do see and treat families have not come out
of the closet. Higher status is associated with individual therapy
than with family therapy. There are a few exceptions, and in such
departments where the family therapist is valued, it is more
likely to be popular with students.

The other major problem about family therapy has to do with
confusion about family and individual therapy. This expresses
itself in concern about who the "identified patient" is. Out of
our traditional responsibility to the person labeled "patient,"
we are still inclined to view the family as ancillary or as blame-
worthy for precipitiating the illness. It may also be regarded as
the source of help and planning for disposition of the "patient"
when treatment is completed. Beginners in family therapy often
carry on one-to-one therapy in the presence of the family, rather
than considering the family as the basic unit of therapy. This
one-to-one approach is extended when the inexperienced therapist
turns from one family member to another, varying the person with
whom the therapy is supposed to be going on, but still maintaining
that it is family therapy since the family is in the room. In
such circumstances the process consists of working with one or
more members of the family, one at a time rather than with the
whole family. The analogy expresses itself in simple things like
records and billing. Our record keeping system is more geared to
individual patients than families. We keep medical records in the
name of the identified patient (the others being listed as
"collaterals") or we open a chart for each individual member of

the family. Rarely or never do we establish a chart for the entire
family. Our colleagues in Family Medicine are beginning to
experiment with family charts. The same is true about billing,
since insurance or other third party schemes assume that a given
person is the unit of illness rather than the entire family.
Similar issues come up around confidentiality, since the "secrets"
of one individual are not kept from other members of the family
in family sessions. Family charts, bills for services to an entire
family, and issues of videotape all bring up concerns about
confidentiality. The therapist must also be willing to decide
when a family member may be seen privately, since such requests
are not infrequent.

Further technical issues center around rooms and spaces. Most
mental health clinic units are established for one-to-one therapy
and offices are built to accommodate two or three people rather
than a whole family. Some centers are experimenting with special
family therapy rooms which include the necessary apparatus for
videotape recordings. Appointments also become an issue when
family therapy is the mode of treatment, since the therapist has
to find a time agreeable to several people, not just to a single
patient.

Students of family therapy may be psychiatrists, psychologists,
social workers and even paraprofessionals. Though there is general
agreement that this is a skill which may be learned by many
disciplines, there is no agreement on the background knowledge or
experience required for learning family therapy. Should each
student be well grounded in individual psychology, including
normal development, psychopathology, and treatment of various disorders? Is family therapy a skill to be primarily devoted to the
mental health settings of clinic or hospital or is it to be
extended to a large variety of family service agencies and other
social service institutions? Another complication associated with
young therapist in training is that they frequently identify with
the young members of the family and are easy prey to the counter-
transference of anti-establishment and anti-parents movement.

ADVANCES REQUIRED FOR THE FIELD--THE TASKS OF THE NEXT DECADE

Though our field has had a brave beginning and has already
influenced the whole field of psychiatry, there are a number of
challenges remaining. It will be necessary for us to develop a
useful classification system for families. If we are to do
research on groups of families, or to develop replicable data on
the most useful approaches to family therapy, we must be able to
describe families. This attempt at classification is basic
to description, to developing an acceptable system of pathology
as well as normality, and is basic to testing the effects of

various interventions. Our reliance on clinical description and anecdotal data has limited the science of families. The increasing breakthroughs in understanding the biology of psychosis may offer opportunities for deeper understanding of the social psychology of families. Studies of communication and family styles give us some hints and have offered some evidence that these efforts can be done reliably.

In part, the challenge of a classification for families relates to the need for a clinically useful theory of family therapy. Beal (1976) contrasts the various schools of family therapy. One group focuses on expression of affect to diminish tension within the family. A contrasting school proposes to create structural change by temporary increase in tension. This permits change in communication pathways or feedback systems. In any clinical discipline, the theory of therapy should be related to understanding functioning, and family therapy should be no different. However, theories of individual psychology are more comprehensive than theories of interaction. For the student who begins a clinical discipline like psychiatry where the focus is on the individual, the jump to family is often managed by assuming that a family is a collection of individuals. Each member of the family is viewed in the same terms as any individual patient who has been studied previously. This avoids the conclusion that the family is a unit of its own with dynamics and developmental problems peculiar to the family. A new psychology, including a theory of therapy, is the point of view needed to truly get the student interested in the family as family--and not as a collection of individual patients.

It is easier to call for more research than to do it. The field has barely gotten well into the hypothesis-generating stage, and most of the research on families lacks systematic design, controls, and the measures to use hypothesis-testing approaches in research. Gurman and Kniskern (1978) have recently reviewed published research in family therapy. They point out that family therapy research often lacks the criteria of replicable and carefully designed studies which attend to sampling, to control for error, to the use of random assignment to different kinds of treatment, and to the use of follow-up and multiple outcome measures. Though some studies are encouraging, they are not well-known to the field. To lend credibility for the student and to encourage further research, training in family therapy should make them more visible. Studies need to be done on the indications for family therapy, differences in outcome (as well as process) from different schools, and to tease out the factors which account for change as a result of family therapy.

Family therapy training is not yet part of every residency

or child fellowship program (Kramer, 1976 and Malone, 1974, 1975).
Indeed, it is not even represented in each program in spite of
the Residency Review Committee requirements. It is not a skill
limited to psychiatry. As a consequence of its newness and its
multidisciplinary base, training in family therapy has often
developed in Family Therapy Institutes rather than traditional
university programs. Family Institutes have been developed by
pioneers in the field who were dissatisfied with the lack of
representation in university programs and they have attracted
students who were already in practice or employed by mental health
agencies (Flomenhaft and Carter, 1977). Though some such
institutes have contributed to child fellowship and general
residency programs, their status outside the university settings
remind us of the institutes which have developed to carry on
psychoanalytic training. However, the differences are considerable
since the psychoanalytic institutes are related to national
professional societies and have organized themselves to enhance
nationally recognized standards. The family therapy institutes
have not achieved a comparable degree of similarity nor have they
achieved the same recognition as has the field of psychoanalytic
training. In spite of the major contributions to education made
by such institutes, one wonders whether this is the most
effective type of organization to promote the incorporation of
family therapy training into recognized programs. These
institutes could be improved by the stability of organized
university programs and stimulated by the fertilization of a
university setting.

REFERENCES

Cuber, J. F. and Harroff, P. B. Sex and the Significant Americans.
    Baltimore:Penguin Books, 1966.
Beal, W. Current trends in the training of family therapists.
    American Journal of Psychiatry, 1976, 133:137-141.
Berman, M. and Leif, H. I. Marital therapy from a psychiatric
    perspective: An overview. American Journal of Psychiatry,
    1975, 132:583-592.
Flomenhaft, K. and Carter, R. Family therapy training: Program
    and outcome. Family Process, 1977, 16:211-218.
Gurman, A. and Kniskern, D.P. Research in marital and family
    therapy:An empirical and conceptual analysis. In:
    S. L. Garfield and A. E. Bergin (Eds.) Handbook of Psycho-
    therapy and Behavioral Change. Second Edition, New York:
    Wiley, 1978.
Kramer, C. Why teach family dynamics and family therapy in a
    general psychiatry residency training program? Family
    Institute, Chicago, 1976, Mimeo, 46 pages.
Lederer, W. and Jackson, D. D. The Mirages of Marriage. New York:
    Norton, 1968.

Liddle, A. and Halpin, J.   Family therapy training and supervision
        literature: A comparative review.   Journal of Marriage and
        Family Counseling, 1978, 4:77-98.
Malone, C. A.   Observations on the role of family therapy in child
        psychiatry training.   Journal of American Academy of Child
        Psychiatry, 1974, 13:437-458.
Malone, C. A.   The family as an integrating focus in basic residency
        training: A case Study.   In L. Madow and C. A. Malone (Eds.)
        The Integration of Child Psychiatry into the Basic Residency
        Program.   Hillsdale, New Jersey:Town House Press, 1975,
        pp. 53-71.

TEACHING FAMILY THERAPY: A DIVISION DIRECTOR'S PERSPECTIVE

Adolph E. Christ, M.D.

Downstate Medical Center-Kings County Hospital

Brooklyn, New York 11203

A Director of a Division of Child and Adolescent Psychiatry juggles a number of priorities. Of these, the most relevant to this symposium are theory-training-service. Each setting has some idiosyncratic service needs, be they the population served, the relative paucity of funds that always results in if-more-for-one-then-less-for-another program, or the interests and expertise of the staff who petition for various training emphases. For example, at Downstate Medical Center-Kings County Hospital the services we provide include an inpatient, a day hospital, an outpatient, a retardation, a child abuse, a sex abuse, a court-adolescent day hospital, a school consultation, a learning disability, a high-risk infant intervention program, and a surgical-pediatric-neurological-and family practice consultation-liaison program. These service obligations are a not unusual list in university-municipal based Divisions.

Similarly, the list of diagnostic procedures and of therapeutic interventions that are required to optimize service and training is also long, and clearly needs to include crisis term and long-term family therapy, individual psychotherapies ranging from psychoanalytically oriented insight oriented to operant conditioning to drug therapy to supportive and environmental altering approaches, not to leave out the various educational and remedial as well as therapeutic milieu approaches. Hence, a multi-diminsional model of psychopathologies and of therapeutic modalities is inescapable.

Whereas, in our situation we have not only the usual university priorities of training and research, but also the municipal hospital with large catchment area priorities of

service, the orientation of a Division is affected. Whereas in
our situation, the majority of referred children have serious
primary or secondary learning problems, ranging from the various
learning disabilities through the subtle to gross basic dysfunction
to the mild to profound retardations, preoccupations for the
emphasis of specific treatments are affected.

Various speakers in this symposium will grapple with the
psychoanalytic single person to the family therapy multi-person
formulations. As a Division Director, despite interest and
experience in family therapy, the University-Municipal Hospital
priorities form an even wider multidimensional perspective.

Using available "theories" as organizing frameworks, rather
than as etiologic theories, can be extraordinarily helpful in
orienting oneself to the vast array of patients and diversity of
their problems with which they come to a child-adolescent psychiatric
center.

Within this multidimensional organizing framework, the psychoanalytic represents one of our essential dimensions. For most
of us, its psychopathological orientation, both in the more
traditional metapsychological and the more recently evolving object
relations perspective, allows us to organize a great deal of the
information we get and generate about our patients. I see the
psychoanalytic perspective as an extremely important and essential
dimension, one that is particularly geared to answer an array of
WHY questions, such as WHY did he behave as he did?

Piaget's concepts of intellectual development, with appropriate
modification[*] provides a second dimension which is particularly
important in organizing information from the more retarded, central
nervous system impaired, psychotic, learning disabled, or other
conflict-free ego impaired individuals. The advantages of Piaget's
theory is that it provides a larger array of developmentally
organized descriptions of intellectual functions. The description
of sequential stages of intellectual organization is particularly
helpful in organizing relevant data generated by our assessments
and interventions with these patients, and is particularly geared
to answer an array of HOW questions, such as HOW (at what stage)
does this person think?

A third complimentary dimension is the neuropsychological
(neurological-neuropathological-neurophysiological) one. This
third dimension is particularly relevant in organizing some

---

*Christ, A. The Clinician's Piaget (in preparation).

information generated by central nervous system damaged, genetically
impaired, learning disabled, severely or profoundly retarded, as
well as many profoundly disturbed individuals. Here, distinctions
between visual and auditory processing difficulties, memory
defects of various types, etc. can be made, distinctions that are
relevant not only in the clearly central nervous system damaged,
but also in many with more subtle and less clear central nervous
system impaired individuals. This framework is particularly
geared to answer WHERE questions, such as WHERE in the brain is
the particular language or memory difficulty organized? Clearly,
all three of these dimensions lend themselves particularly to the
organization of data about a single individual, where the word
INTRAPSYCHIC takes on a more encompassing meaning.

A fourth dimension, and one particularly relevant to this
symposium, is the family or INTERPERSONAL dimension. Whether
one reads Mahler's careful description of the young child's object
relations development through the individuation-separation stage,
Piaget's description of a developmental invariant such as
assimilation-accommodation, or Spitz's descriptions of hospitalism
and anaclitic depression, the importance of the interactional
component in the normal and deviant development is evident. Whether
the emphasis of the family therapist is understanding the effect
of the interaction on each individual in the family using a
psychoanalytic framework, or understanding communicational pathways
or distortions using a cybernetic perspective, or on the family
structure using a systems perspective, or a combination of several
such frameworks, the relevance of thinking family and paying close
attention to the complex interactions of the family in any given
situation that has a disturbed or deviant child or adolescent or
parent is clear. Various speakers in the symposium will describe
what may emerge as helpful organizing frameworks for the rich data
that derives from the study of the family.

A fifth dimension, and one that becomes automatic to individuals
trained in child and adolescent psychiatry and that can serve as a
unifying one for the above four, is the developmental perspective.
Thinking of the interaction of the above four dimensions over time,
but more significantly, during crucial moments in development, can
be helpful. Let us take a 16 month old infant who is in Mahler's
practicing substage of the individuation-separation stage of
development, in Piaget's tertiary circular reaction substage of the
sensorimotor stage of development and which may coincide with a
crucial central nervous development such as the right-to-left
hemisphere shift of function or with pre-frontal or temporal-
parietal-occipital function development, in a family where each
parent encourages and values, or is threatened by early independence,
highlights how the four dimensions may be understood during one
crucial point in development. This dimension is particularly geared
to answer WHEN questions.

Finally, a sixth dimension, one that has been particularly difficult to integrate with the others, is the dimension that allows us to organize meaningfully, information about school, about neighborhood, about social class, about ethnicity, about immigration, about opulent versus decaying neighborhoods, etc. In short, it is all those factors that are larger in scope than individuals or families, yet play a crucial role in the life of the patients and of the families. It is those more socio-economic-cultural parameters to which one of the JANUS-faced perspectives of family interpersonal and individual intrapsychic thinking look. The techniques of social area analysis of a census tract, a health area, a health planning district, a county, city or state, may become useful to provide a way of organizing all this relevant socio-cultural material.

In summary, all six organizing frameworks or perspectives are required to understand the large diversity of patients and situations that present themselves to a large busy child and adolescent psychiatric division. Especially when, as in our situation, the service responsibility is for a diverse social class ethnic catchment area, one strains for ways of understanding the heterogenous problems that require thoughtful intervention. As we try to enlarge the range of patients that may benefit from our involvement, additional organizing frameworks may emerge that will provide the handle that allows our thinking to address the new problems.

THE PLACE OF FAMILY THERAPY IN A DIVISION OF CHILD AND ADOLESCENT PSYCHIATRY

As the Director of a Division in a University setting, one has another dimension of choices one needs to make—these are the training priorities. Clearly, these priorities are of two types. One is the dimension about which treatment modalities to teach and which to emphasize, the second is whether to encourage the teaching of the modalities by highly competent but perhaps zealous specialists, or to choose faculty members interested in the integration of a number of treatment modalities and related theories.

As can be imagined, the types and mixtures of therapeutic modalities that may be required for a setting such as this is large. In addition to the traditional individual, family and group approaches, the large number of ego-impaired and learning disabled children requires at times particular emphasis on tutorial and other psychoeducational techniques, some of the most effective including having a parent learn to tutor, hence requiring a careful assessment of the family dynamic to effect.

It is hard to over-estimate the need for techniques of family

therapy and family intervention. Once one begins to "think family"
it is hard to remember a time when this all pervasive perspective
with requisite modalities was an exception rather than the rule.
A diagnosis of retardation, the interventions with pre-teen rape
or child abuse, a severe school related crisis, a fire or robbery in
the apartment, these and many more require a careful assessment of
the struggles and potential strengths and weaknesses in a family
which may lead to appropriate family related interventions, crisis
family contacts, etc.

As a Director of a multi-modality Division, one can easily
place the Director of Family Therapy in a bind. The only reason
it is not a double bind is that we can at least freely discuss it.
Specifically, I prefer the Director of a therapeutic modality to
be a strong proponent of this modality, to be an expert in it and
enthusiastic about its value so as to infect the trainee with
enthusiasm and so overcome some of the trainee's apprehensions
and initial resistances. On the other hand, given many of the
types of problems that come to a child psychiatry division, not
only are many modalities other than family therapy essential, but a
more free-wheeling combination of individual, family, group, and
other modalities may be required for the same family, concurrently
or alternately. Some family therapy directors prefer to isolate
family therapy, and teach it in a fairly pure form. This allows
a cleaner teaching of specific techniques of family therapy, as
well as specific schools of family therapy thinking. Others prefer
the more eclectic approach, and emphasize that every situation, as
long as it allows the trainee to "think family," is appropriate.

Whichever option is chosen, there is a grave danger that the
trainee can be put into a bind. In such a situation, some trainees
quickly learn to speak differently to different supervisors,
depending upon the supervisors' orientation; others may use this
as a vehicle to goad supervisors. Unfortunately, the smooth
integration of each of the six dimensions is not yet possible, a
task that may have to await the next generation of theoreticians.
Clearly, verbalizing the state of our unintegrated art to the
trainees relieves some of their anxiety, decreases their need to
act out their bind, and may even inspire some to innovative
integrations.

In summary, then, a large division has many treatment
responsibilities that require multidimensional thinking. Similarly,
the need to teach a number of different therapeutic modalities is
clear. There are binds that are inherent in such a multidimensional
approach, binds that have not yet been resolved. Fortunately,
family therapy has taught us that even difficult binds, as long as
they can be talked about, need not necessarily produce pathology.

GAPS IN FAMILY THERAPY PRACTICE: DISCUSSION OF DR. LANGSLEY'S

PAPER

Wells Goodrich, M.D.

Chestnut Lodge

Rockville, Maryland

    Dr. Langsley has raised several major training and clinical
issues with which I resonate strongly. The training of residents,
psychologists, and social workers is very complicated in the
diagnostic treatment planning phase with the disturbed child. How
do you make the choice of whether to go one of three ways:
traditional one-to-one child therapy, family therapy alone, or
concurrent individual and family therapy? This depends partly on
what population you have in the clinic. You may end up, at
least in Rochester where I used to be Head of Child Psychiatry,
with something like 40% or more of the cases initially assigned
to classical one-to-one therapy. Or, do you go the road of an
exploratory initial period with both individual therapy and
concurrent family therapy, while you are getting more deeply
involved in both the understanding of what is going on here and
beginning to make certain initial therapeutic moves? Or, do
you see that individual therapy is really not relevant and you
should start right out with family therapy alone? Until we
conduct more research and follow-up studies, we will not be clear
about the appropriateness and effectiveness of various treatment
strategies.

    We do not have a classification scheme yet for communicating
with each other about the diagnosis of the family. Dr. Langsley
gave us one set of concepts which are fairly familiar. At this
point, each of us has a somewhat different frame of reference.
A few years hence, perhaps, we may be able to do something like
a GAP report and create a family diagnostic scheme that all of us
could use. I find myself employing four overlapping sets of
concepts when I think of family systems. Recently, I received the
criticism, "Gee, you gave a whole talk on family therapy and you

never used the term 'family system'." A primary element of the
family system is the <u>psychoanalytic model</u>, especially the matter
of shared unconscious and conscious conflicts and shared defenses
which are mutually re-enforced between dyads in the family. There
is a second element, the <u>system of roles</u> which is either
inappropriate in terms of boundaries, that is, too close or too
distant, or not functioning appropriately for parent or children.
Family members re-enforcing these roles exhibit patterns and
<u>forms of communication</u>. For example, Lyman Wynne has linked
cognitive style with communication forms as an aspect of individual
ego function. These styles of communication represent family
"ego functions."

   We have a lot of work to do on classification. We are not
going to make further advances in teaching, research or clinical
work until we get that classification. It is a number one priority
for the whole field.

   I feel very concerned personally, as a psychoanalyst and as
a psychotherapist as regards the teaching of individual therapy.
As a by-product of our relative success in community delivery of
brief services at less cost with more modest goals, there has been
an over-reaction in teaching programs leading to a downgrading of
interest and value placed on traditional psychotherapy. Today,
residents are not receiving high quality training in intensive
individual psychotherapy as they would have received 10 or 15
years ago. I think the same problem exists in family therapy now.
One of the things that I particularly resonate with in Dr. Langsley's paper is the need for senior therapists to expose their
work to be viewed by others whether it be individual or family work.
One of the first people I know who systematically did that many
years ago was Rudolf Eckstein, in a regular seminar in front of
the one-way vision screen at Menningers. Once a week, residents
sat and watched him treat a patient in analysis, and then, afterwards, he would discuss his work and they could question him. All
this was done with the permission of the patient. Or, you can
video tape certain selected hours of an advanced therapist for use
in teaching.

   In medical education, compare the situation in psychiatry with
surgery. If you are a resident in surgery, you get direct contact
with the highly seasoned senior surgeon at work. You see how he
operates. You can watch him; you can model on him. After four
or five years of residency in surgery, you realize that there is
still a tremendous lot that you have to learn because you are
working side-by-side this neurosurgeon or this plastic surgeon,
a person who is outstanding as a model and as a teacher.

   I will close by relating an experience which happened to me
this week which illustrates this need for the trainee to join with

more senior clinicians in the work. My role at Georgetown
University is to introduce family therapy into the Division of
Child Psychiatry which had not had family therapy before. I was
asked by a child fellow to do a consultation on a case with which
he was having trouble. We met once with the family last Wednesday.
The fellow had presented the fact that all three children in the
family, age 6, 11, and 17 years, were either passively aggressive
or passively withdrawn. There was a lack of cooperation among
the parents. The father was seen as an aggressive disruptive
force that everyone was afraid of. The mother was seen as a
long-suffering but fairly normally-adjusted peacemaker. Now what
happened when we saw the family was that it was clear that some
of this was true. After a half-hour with the family, it also was
clear that the child psychiatry fellow lacked a sufficient
appreciation of the family. This is the sort of thing that is
sometimes very hard to judge until you have seen a lot of patients.
This mother was, indeed, very schizoid and masochistic. Despite
the smile on her face, and her apparent satisfaction with the way
things were going in the family, there was a total denial of her
own real feelings. She was actually chronically depressed and
helpless, revealing nothing and speaking with very great hesitation
and difficulty about anything. It became clear to me that until
this woman can be helped to be more revealing and understanding
of her own internal feelings, that the whole family is essentially
living with a very, very sick mother. The mother's borderline
psychotic character disorder had been missed by the fellow and by
the staff of the Clinic. I know that sounds self-serving, but I
do think that one's diagnostic skills increase significantly as
a result of years of practice. Clearly, these residents must at
times work directly in the treatment situation with more experienced clinicians.

INTRODUCTION OF FAMILY THERAPY INTO CHILD PSYCHIATRY TRAINING:

TWO STYLES OF CHANGE

Wells Goodrich, M. D.

Chestnut Lodge

Rockville, Maryland

Prior to 1967, I was based at the National Institute of Mental Health for 15 years, and was involved in psychoanalytically-oriented adult psychiatry, child development studies, and family therapy. During the decade following 1967, I spent five years each at two teaching hospitals in New York City[*] and at Rochester, New York.[**] At each of these hospitals, a new family training program was introduced where there had been none previously. Finally, in 1978, I returned to Washington and, for the third time, was asked to introduce family therapy into an ongoing child psychiatry fellowship program at Georgetown University Medical Center. In this paper, I will take the opportunity to reflect upon these three experiences. They illustrate two contrasting styles of introducing family therapy training into training programs in psychiatry, programs which had previously concentrated primarily upon individual diagnosis and therapy.

These two styles of change will be referred to as partial

---

[*]This was Montefiore Hospital (Albert Einstein College of Medicine) in Bronx, New York; the period of time was 1968 to 1971 when Morton Reiser, M. D. was Chairman of that Department of Psychiatry.

[**]The program change discussed here occurred at the University of Rochester Medical Center within the Child and Adolescent Psychiatry Division under my direction and with the active support of the Chairman, Lyman C. Wynne, M.D., Ph.D., and with the assistance of Steven Munson, M.D., Christopher Hodgman, M.D., Roger Shapiro, Ph.D. and Elta Green, M.S.W.

introduction of family therapy versus complete introduction of
family therapy. The complete introduction may be contrasted with
the partial introduction in the following sense: A complete introduction of family therapy training would mean that, following the
change in the program, all patients seen by trainees would routinely have a family diagnostic evaluation and would be considered
for possible family therapy. The trainee would continue to
receive the traditional training in individual diagnosis and learn
indications and considerations for individual therapy. Thus, in
the complete form, the students are taught a both-and approach by
combining family diagnosis and therapy with individual therapy or
with other therapeutic modalities. By contrast, in the partial
introduction, family therapy techniques are considered only as a
special approach for those few selected cases in which obvious
involvement of multiple family members in the individual patient's
pathology makes traditional individual treatment clearly unre-
warding, if not impossible, and for families in which two or more
members are currently symptomatic and in acute need of treatment.
The psychiatric department is not yet ready to employ family
diagnosis routinely in every case, nor is family therapy considered
equally to individual therapy as a possible routine intervention
for all new cases seen in the outpatient clinic or in the hospital.

I should make clear at this point that my own view of these
complex choices is that in selected cases, family diagnosis and
therapy may have much to add to more traditional psychiatric
treatment. The value of the older forms of treatment, such as
group therapy, individual therapy, hospital care, psychopharmacology, etc. have, of course, been proven. Therefore, in all
three experiences of introducing family therapy for the first
time, what I had aimed for was a broadening of the scope of
clinical observation, as well as broadening the number and complexity of therapeutic choices available to the staff and to the
trainees. This orientation introduces greater complexity into
the clinical process. Clinical options and choices involved in
treatment planning become apparent, even for situations for which
no clear-cut guidelines as yet exist. What I refer to here has to
do with criteria for assignment of cases to one or other treatment
modalities at a given stage of a particular form of pathology
either in the individual and/or in the family. Overall, my
impression is that, while a complete introduction of family therapy
has a number of advantages from a theoretical point of view and
should be the ultimate goal of the program change, the style of
starting with partial introduction is administratively easier to
manage and is psychologically much less stressful on faculty.

The ultimate decision for change depends largely on the
conviction and style of the Chairman of the Department. The rapid
changes at Rochester in introducing a much more complete

re-orientation to the training programs were made possible by the strong family orientation and involvement of Lyman Wynne in concert with several full-time faculty already trained in family therapy. These conditions were not present either at Montefiore or at Georgetown to make the more dramatic and theoretically satisfying complete change in the training program.* However, with the passage of time, I find faculty members do become invested in family therapy and gradually approach a more complete change with the partial approach.

A number of paradoxes have become apparent from these three experiences. When a rapid change in the program occurs, the increased scope of therapeutic options augments the treatment effectiveness of the program, but also fosters confusion and disagreement among faculty about which cases to select for which modality. The clinical process tends inevitably to move more toward a treatment team, or at the very least, a co-therapist model, instead of a single therapist model. This facilitates teaching of family diagnosis and therapy, as well as combining of individual therapy concurrently with family therapy. The administrative work, though, is made more complex, and the whole treatment process becomes more prolonged and expensive. A more open intake policy becomes possible for most new admissions to the emergency room or to the clinic. This, however, can burden the trainee's case load with too many difficult character disorders and borderline psychotic patients, while there is an insufficient pool of patients suitable for individual psychoanalytically-oriented psychotherapy.

THE COMPLETE INTEGRATION OF FAMILY THERAPY TRAINING WITH CHILD AND ADOLESCENT PSYCHIATRY TRAINING

The Rochester experience illustrates the achievement of complete integration, something that can realistically only be accomplished when adequate numbers of faculty experienced in all of the major treatment modalities are available at a university-based diverse set of treatment services. We were fortunate in having a departmental chairman who was determined to maintain the excellence of previous training in individual and group therapy, but who also wished to introduce both family therapy and behavior modification in an integrated fashion to the training programs in child and adult psychiatry. This necessitated revising and making

---

*The partial changes were introduced (within my experience) at the Montefiore Hospital general psychiatric residency; at Georgetown University in Washington and at Rochester, New York. The complete style of introduction was carried out within the child and adolescent psychiatry program.

more complex the previously existing service delivery systems in
the clinics and in the hospital, as well as making the training
programs more differentiated. Work was increased in geometric
proportion for the administration of the training programs,
since both the number and the complexity of decisions increased
with respect to treatment planning options for the patients, to
assignment of trainees to cases, and to supervision of trainees.

When one to three family interviews are required for all
evaluations on new patients, a whole range of previously unnoticed
clinical data emerges. These new facts reveal new clinical
syndromes which have to be considered in treatment planning and
in the assignment of the case to the students who may or may not
be technically ready to provide the required service. In addition,
supervisors have to be available who have the expertise to
recognize and respond to such family systems data. These clinical
syndromes include: (1) family developmental stage disturbances;
(2) family stress syndromes; and, (3) long-term structural
abnormalities of the family which have their origins in psychodynamic genetic processes, in chronic role dysfunctions, and in
chronic patterns of inadequate family communication.

(1) Family developmental stage disturbances. Notwithstanding
the diagnosis, the acutely disturbed adolescent patient can be
understood as responding to parents whose anxieties lead them to
vacillate between being overly close (seductive) versus being
overly distant or punitive. Often, one of the parents has stepped
out of appropriate parental role functioning and is behaving more
like a sibling. On the other hand, the parent may have difficulties
with control issues, either failing to set limits for the adolescent, setting too rigid controls, or both at different times.
These dysfunctional parent-child relationships interfere with the
adolescent's emancipation process from the family. The problem of
early adolescent depression and/or rebellion which is out of
control may arise from similar family circumstances and lead to
an over-identification with an antisocial peer group. At an
earlier age, school phobia problems of recent onset in a 5 to 7
year old may involve neurotic anxieties shared between child and
mother. These situations reflect the family struggling to move
from one stage of development to another which can best be resolved
with family therapy.

(2) Family stress syndromes. With increasing frequency, one
sees children from the post-divorce family and the family
disrupted by the death of one parent. In the post-divorce process,
families often need help in setting up new parental and new child
roles, when a step-parent is brought into the family or when
children from two previously established families are amalgamated
as step-siblings into a new family structure. As a result of not

having completed the mourning process, the remaining single parent
sometimes unconsciously utilizes one of the children as a
substitute spouse. This unconscious pathological alliance between
parent and child may require attention through a family approach
before the parent can again observe appropriate parent-child role
boundaries and before the child can be free to invest in a more
appropriate adaptation.

(3) Long-term family structural abnormalities. In families,
structural problems of a psychopathological nature may be
illustrated by chronic triangulation or scapegoating of one child
as a displacement from covert marital problems which parents have
been unwilling or unable to face and resolve for many years. As
an intermediate clinical intervention, family therapy may be
useful when one senses that the family can initially accept help
only for the "disturbed child." Family therapy may provide needed
support to the scapegoated child by re-establishing parent-child
boundaries. A preliminary period of family therapy may be required
to assist the parents develop sufficient trust in the clinicians
to begin to reveal and discuss the underlying marital conflict.
Then, at a later stage, the couple may be able to accept a shift
from family to marital therapy.

In the Rochester experience, where many clinicians are
experienced in and available for the application of several
modalities, and when routine family diagnosis is applied with all
children who are evaluated, I found that 20 to 30 percent of
cases will be assigned to a combination of individual child therapy
plus concurrent family therapy as an initial treatment plan. This
still left 40 percent of the cases to be assigned to individual
therapy, as might have occurred more routinely prior to the introduction of family therapy. A small percentage was assigned to
group therapy or behavior modification.

Treatment planning has to consider what is acceptable to the
family. In a significant minority of cases, a treatment approach
may be initiated to engage the family, although it does not
represent what the clinician favors. Rather, that may be the only
approach that the family will accept at the outset. The treatment
service is based on the assumption that, over time, many family
members will move from individual to family treatment and from
family to individual treatment, or through other treatment
modalities as family or individual defenses shift and new problems
emerge or old problems are solved.

CONCEPTUAL ORIENTATIONS TO FAMILY THERAPY

Within the domain of family therapy, it is useful to conceptualize four theoretical and technical styles of family work.

Each one of the approaches analyzes different aspects of disturbed
family functioning, involves different foci of therapeutic intervention, and has developed a unique body of literature. All
four conceptual orientations can be applied within a family and
in an individual developmental frame of reference.

Among these four orientations, the broadest and most integrative frame of reference is the psychoanalytic with its focus on
needs, affects, perceptions, and fantasies in relationship with
its constant monitoring of defenses and conflicts. Conflicts
and defenses are recognized as either conscious or unconscious,
as well as individual or shared among family subsystems.

The second frame of reference is family role structure, which
has been derived from cultural anthropology and social psychology.
The clinical applicability of this frame of reference has been
cogently taught by Minuchin (1974). This approach is more quickly
grasped by new trainees than the psychoanalytic one, and often
provides at least a temporary sense of therapeutic movement and
progress. Analyzing family disorders in terms of dysfunctional
parent-child roles highlights family role boundaries, overly rigid
role functioning, and problems in parental decision-making. When
family role behavior is being modified, anxiety is mobilized and
new defenses will emerge. The therapy challenges long-standing
family structures in the intrapsychic defenses of the family
members. Thus, hidden conflicts within each family member need
to be explored and understood before prominent role changes can
take place. In this process, the family therapist may be alerted
to the need for individual psychotherapy for formerly nonsymptom-
atic family members. As part of this process, symptoms sometimes
may shift from the patient to be assumed by other family members.

A third set of concepts focuses upon distortions in the
process of family communication, which has been found useful to
guide family and marital therapy. This frame of reference has
been particularly applicable in clinical settings (family social
service agencies, educational counseling services, marital
counseling centers) providing services to the less seriously ill.
Even when treating more disturbed psychiatric patients, and when
employing primarily a psychoanalytic or family role centered focus,
attention by the therapist to the disturbed communication process
in their families will be a useful part-process within the total
therapeutic approach. The therapist will actively interrupt
inappropriate modes of communication, confront family members with
repetitive types of communication that need to be relearned, and
demonstrate the ways that dysfunctional communication leads to
misunderstanding and misperception among family members. The
effort here is toward greater clarity in self-expression and more
accurate interpersonal perception. The therapist strives to attain
clear definitions of individual realities and of the shared family

reality. The family members are repeatedly confronted with their
ambiguity, incompleteness, or fragmentation of communication.
Attempts are made to reduce behaviors such as ignoring one another
or interrupting one another. Interpreting the meaning of what
another family member is saying as being quite different than what
was actually said or intended, is stopped by the therapist who
urges the family members to listen and to accept the messages
actually communicated. Particularly in impulse-ridden families,
who may bring a delinquent child for treatment, a great deal of
work may have to be done simply in retraining the family toward
more appropriate modes of communication before more fundamental
treatment goals such as change in family roles or insight into
underlying unconscious conflicts can be addressed.

The fourth frame of reference is that of behavior modification
as a form of family therapy. Behavior modification is relevant
to the family therapist primarily as it contributes to a greater
understanding of learning processes which are to be found as a
part process within all forms of psychotherapy. In practice,
behavior modification provides a way of utilizing the parents as
therapeutic aides to assist the therapist in bringing about
changes in the behavior of one or more of the children. Particularly in children who have limited symptomatology and who live
in a family with considerable ego strength, the behavior modification
approach may be an efficient way of facilitating healthy adaptation
of children at a particular developmental stage.

In my own work and in the work of many faculty colleagues of
my acquaintance, the major frame of reference for family therapy
work is the psychoanalytic which has the broadest scope to
integrate the concepts of family communication, role dysfunction,
and learning theory. This focus, however, on psychodynamically-
oriented family therapy has to be recognized as quite different
in style from traditional individual psychodynamic psychotherapy.
Even though there is a focus on the complex interplay among family
members of needs, conflicts, and defenses (including projections
and various forms of maladaptive relationships), the style of the
therapist's work is much more active than in psychoanalytic
individual work. Since family systems are extremely rigid and can
work against the therapist's wish to make changes, the therapist
needs an active stance which encourages family members to initiate
new ways of relating to each other by trial and error. This is
done early as maladaptive forms of relationships are identified
and clarified within the family sessions. Thus, one moves rapidly
from demonstrating inappropriate and maladaptive patterns of family
experience and behavior into efforts to change these patterns toward
more appropriate styles of relating. As Minuchin (1974) has
pointed out, even when this serves to mobilize further struggles
rather than to allay conflict, much is learned through attempts
at new and more appropriate ways of relating. The mere fact that

families can begin to recognize the undesirability of their own habitual ways of relating, the defensive functions of these patterns will further motivate members toward new observations and new insights into the specific nature of the underlying conflicts which are shared among the family members.

The whole process of family therapy is made possible by an initial phase in which the family therapist becomes psychologically identified as a temporary family member and experiences directly the cross-currents of family conflict and defense. The family therapist's own counter-transference reactions can be most useful as indicators of hidden images, myths, legends, and misperceptions. The layering of defenses and conflicts means that when one issue is resolved, then a new layer of formerly unobservable defense and conflict becomes expressed. This repeats for the clinician what he has earlier observed to happen in individual work with patients.

THE TEACHING MODEL

The training program addresses three large groups of trainees: (a) medical students or first year psychiatric residents who are simply being oriented to the nature of clinical observation and to the clinical process with children and adolescents; (b) child-fellows who are at a mid-phase; or (c) at a more advanced phase of learning about psychiatry. Suitable training experiences, supervision, not to mention acquaintance with available literature and other aspects of the curriculum, naturally need to be quite different depending upon the degree of clinical experience of the trainee. The nature of cases which can be accepted into a training clinic for treatment depends in good part upon the ratio of advanced to beginner trainees in the program at any one time. From the point of view of providing service to the patients, it is well to have an approximately equal number of students at various levels of competence in the clinic at any one time. In many university settings, it is not feasible to have faculty members carry a heavy case load because of their teaching responsibilities, nor is it usually financially possible to have a large backup clinical staff to supplement the work of trainees. Therefore, at certain times of the year, when teaching programs are coming to an end or when an influx of new trainees is expected, temporary waiting lists have to be employed where cases can be kept on reserve for as much as one or two months in order to fit the treatment processes into the available therapeutic competence levels of trainees.

BEGINNING LEVEL

At the beginning level, the students need to focus on basic

family interviewing techniques and learn the major diagnostic
syndromes. The initial tasks are learning to develop a therapeutic alliance and to form an initial treatment plan. These
are best accomplished by the student observing more experienced
students or faculty. After having observed others for several
weeks, and after having received a didactic preparation, the
student's work in family therapy is often best initiated using the
co-therapy approach. Here, the co-therapist may be either an
advanced child psychiatry fellow who serves as an instructor for
the raw beginner, or a faculty member. A new case is taken on
in family therapy which is appropriate for co-therapy, and, in the
initial experience of this sort, the student plays a relatively
passive role. When the student has gained confidence and finds
that he has achieved an effective therapist role along with the
more senior co-therapist, he may wish to begin a family without
a partner. Throughout this initial phase of training, the one-way
mirror is of particular value. We have tried to use a more active
monitoring technique, such as the bug-in-the-ear, and found this
somewhat distracting for trainees. However, with the beginning
family therapy trainee, the work needs to be very carefully
monitored. Most sessions should be observed directly by the
supervisor and not simply videotaped for later playback. The
reason for this is that the range of crisis situations which can
arise for a relatively untrained beginning family therapist with
a new family situation is great and cannot always be anticipated.
In the early family sessions, situations often arise requiring
immediate therapeutic action combined with firmness and tact in
order to save the therapeutic alliance and to avoid losing the
family. Thus, the student and the family are both prepared for
the possibility of being interrupted in the middle of a session
either by the faculty member knocking on the door, or by the use
of a telephone communication system into the interview room from
the observation booth. This can be managed tactfully and
supportively with the family, provided the family is prepared
in advance for these possibilities. Obviously, this kind of
intensive supervision for the beginning family therapist can only
be provided where there are adequate numbers of faculty available
who are widely experienced with family psychopathology. Thus,
to implement this approach with more than a very small number of
students (that is to say, to implement it as a routine training
procedure for all those who are taking training in child and
adolescent psychiatry) is not feasible in the partial introduction
mode which we have referred to above. It is only possible at a
stage in a training program in which family therapy is routinely
available and in which family diagnosis is part of the routine
work-up on all new child cases.

INTERMEDIATE LEVEL

    For the intermediate level of traineeship, the supervisor
needs to review substantially all the work which has occurred
in the previous week on a week-by-week basis. This is only
practical by the use of classical verbal retrospective recording
from notes, with only occasional use of individual videotape
playback for supervision. Students at the intermediate level will
be reading more advanced literature, will be attending a group
supervision of a videotape of one of their student colleagues and
will be receiving a large amount of close supervision.

ADVANCED LEVEL

    The more advanced levels of traineeship require proportion-
ately less time of the faculty members, since the student has
reached a level of considerable experience. Videotape playback
can be used both in individual and small group supervision. The
focus of videotape or other retrospective review of therapeutic
work is on details of interactions in the therapeutic situation.
Thus, it is virtually impossible, using videotape, to review each
week the entire scope of the previous week's work. Supervision
tends to focus on a very small portion of the previous week's
session. Faculty can comfortably permit the student to carry a
large number of families in family therapy without close monitoring
and with supervision limited to issues which are largely selected
by the student himself. Of course, periodic review, such as
every one to three months, of all the advanced student's work, is
necessary to continue to insure quality of service as well as
excellence of training.

TRAINING FACULTY TO ASSUME ROLES IN FAMILY THERAPY EDUCATION:
PARTIAL APPROACH

    Where family therapy training is introduced in the partial
approach, faculty competence is enhanced by including interested
members in a didactic seminar plus small group supervision of
family therapy cases. These are best presented at first to
advanced child psychiatry fellows plus one or two potentially
interested faculty. Case material is selected carefully to
generate enthusiasm for a wider application of family therapy
services and training. After six months to a year, faculty
members, as well as advanced child psychiatry fellows, will begin
to undertake more family therapy cases and to obtain wider
experience with less close supervision.

    By the second year of the "partial approach," it is

important to have both a beginning weekly group supervision seminar
as well as an advanced group supervision seminar. The beginning
family therapy seminar will be maintained for those who have not
had previous experience in family therapy and eventually may be
open to first year child psychiatry fellows. The purpose of the
advanced group supervision seminar is to consider more difficult
technical issues such as counter-transference, choice of intervention techniques within a particular videotaped sequence, etc.
The focus of the beginner's group supervision seminar is on more
elementary issues, such as methods for obtaining an initial working
contract with the family or on techniques for dealing with family
defenses in the initial phase of a new case. Whereas the advanced
seminar may focus on the issues of the middle or termination phases
of family therapy, the beginner's seminar tends to focus on the
early phases of treatment.

Eventually, however, there will be a need for a third kind
of seminar with the increasing numbers of trained faculty persons
supervising family therapy within the child psychiatry program.
This is for faculty members who may have taught child psychiatry
for years, but who have never taught family therapy before. Its
focus is to share their dilemmas and questions with one another.
The faculty supervision seminar can show videotapes of the supervisory sessions, always, of course, with the permission of the
students. Gradually, as time passes, evaluation by the students
of the faculty, as well as the evaluations of the students by
the faculty, become built into the training program. Workshops
led by outside leaders in the field of family therapy can be
arranged to stimulate the introduction of new concepts and
techniques both to faculty members and to trainees.

COMPLETE APPROACH

In the complete introductory mode of changing the program
radically within a short period of time, a great many operational
changes must take place within a few weeks or months. The introduction of so many changes (for the faculty and trainees at all
levels and for the advanced trainees, as well as for the faculty
members who are beginning to teach family therapy for the first
time) add up to a considerable degree of institutional stress.
The advantage of the rapid introduction of an ambitious set of
changes is that it is possible for the benefits of family therapy
to be demonstrated clinically with the patients, as well as
educationally with the students. Also, if there are institutional
reasons for a major program change in order to demonstrate the
progressive nature of the department of psychiatry, there may be
a great deal of motivation among the faculty group to carry out
such widespread changes rapidly. As indicated earlier, this is,
of course, only feasible where four to six faculty members are

available to support all of these new undertakings. Where the
faculty has expressed concern about the absence of family therapy
in the past, a lively faculty seminar has emerged. After the first
few meetings, this group reduced itself in number from the initial
70 to about 20 or 25 faithful attending faculty members. These,
then, later contributed to a roster of available supervisors for
work with fellows and students in child and in adult psychiatry
who were learning family therapy.

ADMINISTRATIVE CHANGES IN THE CLINIC INTAKE PROCESS

The initial judgment about the degree to which family psychopathology forms an intrinsic component of the child's own disorder,
as contrasted with the child who has developmentally internalized
intrapsychic conflicts and is no longer deeply affected by the
family conflicts, is an extremely difficult one. Often, judgments
have to be made largely on the basis of intuition and personal
clinical "feel." Thus, by the time the data from the first few
family and individual interviews have been gathered, with the
appropriate laboratory examinations and/or psychological tests,
there remain many unanswered questions which confront the
administrator responsible for case assignment and for treatment
planning. While these decisions can be delegated to a senior
clinician experienced in both individual and family therapy
modalities, the training program benefits greatly from having
these decisions reviewed and discussed each week by a senior
faculty committee made up of those faculty who carry the major
teaching responsibilities for all of the child psychiatry training
programs. Committee members have a valuable opportunity to
confront each other with the many intriguing and vital questions
about the diagnosis of child and family psychopathology, degree
of family psychopathology, issues of prognosis and tactics in
management. The initial judgment must be made as to whether the
family approach or the individual approach makes more sense.
After three to six months in the clinic, a review of treatment
can provide a healthy check on these predictions and evaluations.
Ideally, a follow-up study six to 12 months after termination of
treatment should also be part of the clinic's routine procedure
and lend further checks on the accuracy of the original predictions.

The faculty conferences that are concerned with case assignment and treatment planning constitute the best internal administrative review of the whole complex interplay between clinic
services and training programs. Conflicts among the needs of the
trainees, the needs of the patients, and the needs of the faculty
inevitably emerge most visible at the moment of decision between
various treatment modalities for a given family or a patient.
The questions raised in such meetings can stimulate faculty
members to undertake clinical studies or to review theoretical or

technical therapeutic papers from the literature to present to
each other.

At the present state of our knowledge, no matter how
experienced the director of the clinic may be, I believe that
no expert anywhere has the total knowledge that is ultimately
going to be needed in clinical child psychiatry. At least two
or three decades of clinical research lies ahead. These studies
must include follow-up studies and many comparative studies of
similar cases assigned to different treatment modalities, followed
up with quantitative indices of improvement or failure. Until
these studies have been done, and they are only now beginning to
be done, the many fascinating questions about the course of child
psychiatric illness and the course of treatment at various developmental stages for various diagnostic groups remain unanswered.
Considering our lack of sure and certain knowledge, faculty
members need to be supported administratively to live with these
ambiguities. More traditional and conservative faculty members
will naturally find this situation rather stressful and may wish
to limit their teaching role to one or another segment of the
training program within which they can operate with less ambiguity.
Thus, certain faculty members may wish only to supervise those
cases that have been found appropriate for family therapy. Other
faculty members may wish to limit their teaching to classical
analytically-oriented individual therapy or behavior modification,
depending on their own professional orientation. In the end,
however, the integration of teaching individual and family therapy
depends upon having a core group of faculty members who are
invested in both approaches to child psychopathology, and who
can sustain a fascination with the many unknowns consequent to
a concurrent investment in both therapeutic approaches.

OVERVIEW--PARTIAL VERSUS COMPLETE STYLE OF INTRODUCING FAMILY
THERAPY INTO CHILD PSYCHIATRY TRAINING

As we have already seen, the departmental situation will,
in good part, determine how gradually or how rapidly the ultimate
goals of introducing family therapy training into child psychiatry
programs can be implemented. Much depends upon the motivation
of the leadership among the faculty and the experience of faculty
members with individual and family therapy. This will in turn
determine their readiness to support rapid changes in the training
program. Not until a significant portion of the faculty members
or the top leadership of the department have had extensive
experience with the limits as well as the practical advantages of
family therapy, will a real change be possible.

The experiences reviewed in this paper reveal that there
are both advantages and disadvantages to either approach to change

a training program. The partial introduction of family therapy
through a specialty seminar has the decided advantage of not
rocking the boat within the department. Awareness of the
applicability of family therapy, as well as its limits, unfolds
gradually among the trainees and faculty as clinical work is
reported upon with illustrative families. A gradual change follows
over several years with the expansion of awareness about the
applications of family therapy among faculty members and trainees.
As a result, administrative values change, and the bases for
administrative decisions and priorities begin to change within
the department. One disadvantage of this partial approach to
change is that for a long time only a limited range and variety
of cases are treated. The entire range of application for family
therapy is not seen under these circumstances. The intake
selection criteria for the university services tend to be too
limited since the potentials of family therapy to meet the needs
for treating the difficult case have not yet been realized. The
increased ability of the university service to participate in the
real world of community services is restricted more than it would
be in situations where family therapy is widely accepted and
practiced in the service delivery system. Another disadvantage
of the gradual approach to change is that it provides more
opportunities for institutionalized resistances to family therapy,
resistance based usually on the anxious fantasies of the more
conservative faculty members. The actuality of both the
advantages and the difficulties of the family therapy field may
thus not be confronted in reality.

     Similarly, the more radical and complete style of introducing
family therapy as a healthy competitor for the individual approach
also brings with it both gains and losses. The overriding
advantage is that everyone involved in the service comes to be
able to see the application of both individual and family therapy
to a large variety of cases. Whole syndromes in which family
therapy can be demonstrated to be particularly effective can be
observed, recalled, and informally collected in one's mind. This
removes the limitation of seeing family therapy as a special
approach, and permits faculty and trainees to consider all of the
potential applications for family therapy. If taken seriously,
the administrative processing at intake becomes broadened and
cases which would have formerly been rejected can now be accepted.
These positive changes, however, are not without their drawbacks.
Rapid changes may mobilize faculty anxiety which may lead to
subgroup formation for and against family therapy. Certain
faculty inevitably become identified more as family therapy
supervisors and others as more individual therapy supervisors,
unless faculty members work hard to balance their own teaching
and treatment investments between these two modalities. A certain
level of competition grows up among the various treatment modalities. This may provide a healthy stimulus for academic study and

investigation, provided it does not lead to unpleasant political
by-products. Administratively, things become considerably more
difficult since the goals of all training programs now become
more complex. The didactic curriculum becomes longer and more
varied, and the monitoring of various kinds and levels of
competence of trainees becomes considerably more complex. More
is expected of the advanced trainee in terms of competence. Paradoxically, with all of this, there is an increased need for
full-time social workers and other clinical staff to back up the
training program. Since the intake process tends to be less
restrictive, the service load tends to accumulate more difficult
cases. This has the advantage of providing a more realistic
atmosphere within the university services for seeing the full range
of difficult cases, but may add to the financial and administrative
burdens of running a service for teaching purposes.

CONCLUSION

This presentation is based upon the clinical view that there
are core therapies and that there are specialized therapies within
child and adolescent psychiatry. Family therapy and individual
therapy, which are carried out in a manner consistent with psychoanalytic principles and which are enriched by other views of the
family as noted above, should be available to all who seek child
psychiatric services. I believe that either therapeutic approach
alone or in some combination may be needed in most cases to
provide adequate assistance to our patients. There is a wide
range of clinically significant questions which remain to be dealt
with by our field, and which have to do with how decisions are
made in applying these two modalities in relation to each other.
The other modalities of treatment with their established uses,
principles, and techniques, should be considered as specialty
therapies. I have reference here to the use of child groups,
adolescent talking groups or adolescent activity groups, behavior
modification, parent counseling, multifamily groups, and the use
of psychopharmacology. A relatively smaller proportion of patients
may best be assigned to these specialized therapies. Often,
these special therapeutic approaches can most usefully be applied
after an initial exploratory phase of diagnostic work which
employs some combination of family and individual therapy. This
paper addresses questions related to how one can move a child
and adolescent training program from being exclusively individual-
therapy-centered to a program combining family therapy and individual therapy on an equal basis in training and in service
delivery.

On the basis of the above experiences, let us consider the
situation of an established department of psychiatry (not undergoing major changes in faculty composition and faculty leadership)

which wishes to add family therapy as a new modality of treatment
and of training. A gradual set of changes seems to make the most
sense to me. Considering the fact that in the end we are talking
about a rather comprehensive change in all three levels of
departmental functioning--the service delivery system, the training
programs, and the competence and organization of faculty--it seems
wise to allot at least three or four years to these change
processes. The issues to be dealt with in bringing about these
changes are many, and include the professional values and clinical
perceptions among the departmental leadership and the faculty.
One needs also to take into consideration the available number
of consultants or faculty who are ready to undertake teaching in
family work and to take clinical responsibility for the services
that must be provided. The number of beginning trainees who,
ultimately, will have to receive supervision in family therapy--
supervision which will have to be very close during the early
weeks of their work with families--needs to be gauged. Another
factor which needs to be monitored is the number of new faculty
available at a given time who may wish to add family supervision
as a new role. Have they reached enough comfort and competence
in their own work with families to begin to provide adequate
supervision? A key factor which interacts with the previous ones
is the degree of openness in the intake process of the various
services provided by the child and adolescent psychiatry group.
The degree to which those patients are accepted into the service
system, particularly those who require family approach, has to be
reviewed from time to time. For example, if the intake system is
opened up to difficult multiproblem families, financially troubled
families, families with intractable psychosomatic illness, or if
the service delivery system attempts to provide a lot of family
crisis intervention, then a very large number of both trained
faculty and trainees in the processes of learning about family
therapy will be required. As the openness for intake of such
families does increase, the trainees and faculty have to be
available and ready. It is most useful, of course, to have a
group of social workers or other clinical personnel without
training responsibilities available to provide services outside
the training program. They provide backup service roles where the
meshing of trainees, faculty and patients work out with an excess
of patients who need to be taken care of.

Finally, I would suggest as a model, a five-step process for
these changes in a training program:

(1) First, a period of time providing a didactic seminar
plus a small group supervision for beginning family therapy
training. These two seminars should initially admit only advanced
child psychiatry trainees and motivated faculty members.

(2) After the above has been successful for a period of time

and has received support from the department, it will be necessary to add a third seminar for advanced-level family therapy technique. This will include those faculty members who eventually will become supervisors. This seminar addresses itself to difficult moments in the process of long-term family therapy, in contrast to the beginning family therapy seminar, which deals with issues of diagnosis and treatment planning and the early moves in family therapy technique.

(3) When sufficient faculty have been trained, a faculty supervisor's meeting is useful for a number of purposes. It helps the faculty to learn from each other. It helps to build faculty morale around the use of the new family therapy modality. And, it helps as a forum for discussion of difficult problems and supervision of the trainees.

(4) Once the faculty manpower have been made available through these processes, or through hiring outside faculty to join the department, a specialty family therapy clinic may be a useful interim procedure as part of the service delivery system. This is not recommended as a permanent entity, however, since it still serves to maintain the specialty status of family therapy. However, as a demonstration clinic for the department to see what family therapy can do for the total service delivery system, it has a temporary usefulness en route to the goal of the development of a more complete system.

(5) After several years, it is hoped that sufficient change in perceptions and values in the department will have taken place, so that the specialty family clinic can be discontinued and an integrated intake and evaluation system can be applied for all child and adolescent cases with all cases receiving both individual and family diagnostic appraisal. All cases will, thereby, receive a balanced consideration for both modalities in all treatment planning. As mentioned before, this will require that there will be approximately equal numbers of faculty in the department trained in family work and in individual work, and that there must be a significant proportion of faculty who are equally comfortable and interested in both modalities. The aforementioned three levels of training seminars should be maintained: (1) the didactic and clinical supervision seminars for beginners, (2) the supervision meetings for the advanced trainees and (3) the faculty supervision meetings which serve to maintain and to elaborate standards both for service and for training.

REFERENCES

Minuchin, S. Families and Family Therapy. Cambridge, Mass.:
    Harvard University Press, 1974.

A DISCOURAGING DESCRIPTION OF INTRODUCING FAMILY THERAPY IN AN INSTITUTION: DISCUSSION OF DR. GOODRICH'S PAPER

Henry Grunebaum, M.D.

Harvard Medical School

Cambridge, Massachusetts

Dr. Goodrich has given us an excellent description of the two major ways that family therapy training can get introduced into psychiatric training. I want to delineate three main influences that impact on this change:

(a) There is the administrative and financial support that is available and the commitment to it of the training director and the person in charge of the institution.

(b) It will be influenced by the population of patients being served and the commitment of the institution to that population.

(c) It will be determined by certain aspects of the ideology of the institution.

Since most of this is spelled out in our paper which will follow this afternoon, I will not deal with these issues at the moment. Rather, I will review the early history of our field and describe the introduction of family therapy into an institution where it had never been thought of, and which the administration was variously indifferent, at best, and mildly hostile at worst.

In the early 60s, a group of staff and residents of the Massachusetts Mental Health Center began to be interested in working with whole families and formed a study group for this purpose. Among the members were Norman Paul, Richard Chasin, Martell Bryant, Jack Weltner, Michael Seltzer and myself. Our motivations were various. Some of us were dissatisfied with the effectiveness of current approaches to schizophrenia. Others were interested in

the mother-child relationship, particularly, as seen in joint
admission. Others were simply curious about what could be learned
by studying the whole family. In retrospect, I am impressed how
little reading we did and how much we went off on our own to
learn what we could from the patients. Perhaps, we were not merely
rebelling against the prevalent ideology of the hospital, but
also against other authorities. The study group attempted to
interview at least one family a week together, and some members
soon began to work with whole families.

There was considerable administrative concern about "wild
family therapy without supervision" when in fact, it was the
case of the lame leading the blind. However, the administration
was also reassured by the fact that the only patients being seen
in this curious form of therapy were viewed as untreatable by
the rest of the staff. If we were going to do harm, at least
the people being harmed were probably hopelessly ill at best. I
suspect new therapies are often tolerated when attempted with
the sickest patients, whether or not this turns out to be the
optimal group for that form of therapy in the end.

After one year of meetings, the study group continued but,
in addition, family diagnostic interviewing became a routine
procedure on two of the wards where the staff members Paul and
Grunebaum and the residents Bryant and Chasin were in charge.
These practices continued as long as these staff members were in
charge of these wards, but ceased as soon as they left for other
positions. There then was a divergence of interest in the group.
Residents left to pursue their own careers elsewhere. Dr. Paul
felt strongly that family evaluation should be routine, and every
resident should learn to do family therapy, an example of
Dr. Goodrich's complete style of introduction. This view was
clearly not compatible with the administration of the hospital,
and Dr. Paul soon left for other more rewarding work. I, on the
other hand, stayed and was gradually able to interest a few members
of the staff in family therapy in the outpatient department and
teaching family evaluations on the inpatient services.

In large measure, this gradual introduction of family therapy
depended on the benign neglect of the administration, which was
willing to tolerate changes that occurred slowly and added to,
but did not attempt to replace or threaten the primary thrust of
the training. But even this partial introduction of family
therapy ended when a new director was appointed with other
interests and placed his own appointees in charge of family therapy
training which became more psychoanalytic in focus, an orientation
which was clearly more compatible with the general ideology of
the hospital. Thus, one gifted trainee who was very interested
in family therapy and had a particular gift for the structural

approaches was initially appointed to a junior position and then
not re-appointed.

This is not a particularly encouraging story, but it does
illustrate the vicissitudes of the introduction of new theories
to institutions. Doubtless, pioneers in this field such as Murray
Bowen, Nathan Ackerman, Israel Zwerling and countless others who
have attempted to influence the practice of institutions have
similar stories to tell and similar scars to show. The experience
is not unique to family therapy, however, and applies equally well
to other theories and therapies.

What conclusions are we to draw from these experiences?
Perhaps it is that institutions may be directed by individuals who
will tolerate many and conflicting ideologies and practices, by
others who will attempt to integrate various ideologies into a
coherent whole which may or may not leave out some, and finally,
directors who will pick and choose narrowly what they will
tolerate. Institutions have histories and often forget their
own past rapidly. What can be accomplished in them will depend
on the climate of the times.

Today, fortunately, the times are ripe for the teaching of
family therapy and for family therapists. But what should family
therapists be asking ourselves? Probably we should ask what are
the therapies and theories of the future? Who are we excluding
at the moment? And, we should think of attempting to foster
their development as we would wish our own to have been fostered.
Thank you.

DO YOU RECOMMEND FAMILY THERAPY OR INDIVIDUAL THERAPY? GENERAL

DISCUSSION

DR. CHRIST

Thank you very much Dr. Grunebaum. Are there any questions or comments?

AUDIENCE MEMBER

One of the decisions to be made in evaluating a patient is whether to recommend individual or family treatment. There is, however, a more primary question. What kind of overall theory are we going to work under, psychoanalytic theory or systems theory? In your response, could you also comment on the process of change?

DR. GOODRICH

I am very pleased that you are raising these issues which need further clarification. I am not talking about psychoanalytic technique of having one patient in the office, rather, psycho-analytic concepts as elements in family systems theory. Family systems theory came from physics, and, originally referred to the elements of feedback loops and certain kinds of change processes which originally were discovered in physics. A lot of the early research was done by the Bell Telephone Laboratories. The notion of a system with formal properties refers to feedback systems and shared resonating systems between different elements. You can put whatever concepts into that that you wish, it is simply a form. It is true that a lot of the people who, in the early days pushed the words family systems were actually interested in communication and role concepts and were rebelling against analytic thinking. In my work as an analyst who likes to teach both individual therapy and family therapy, I find such notions as two people in the family sharing a defense, and reinforcing the same denial and the same projection against, perhaps, a very similarly shared unconscious conflict to be the central aspect of my way of using the concept family systems.

Now the theory of change is something that is an important question which I did not address. The question is puzzling. If you just do family therapy, it could be put this way: Are you simply creating role change? Perhaps there is some shift in defenses in certain members, resulting in better adaptation among family members, calling on ego resources in each member as they help to support each other, clarifying reality, behaving more appropriately with each other, and finally, experiencing each other more realistically and empathically. Or, are you actually creating as a by-product, perhaps, some "intrapsychic structural change" as an aspect of an outcome of family therapy? I do not know the answer. It seems to me that the work of individual therapy is more explicitly oriented towards intrapsychic change, and the work of family therapy is more explicitly oriented towards interpersonal structure. These are tough questions.

AUDIENCE MEMBER

At the institution where I trained, the senior family therapy teachers and the senior analytic teachers could not talk to each other. If you went to a family therapy class and you mentioned the word anxiety or unconscious, that was an automatic "F". What I find happening is that clinical decisions are based on your orientation to human behavior. If you are analytic, you make analytically oriented dispositions; if you are family therapy oriented, you make family therapy oriented decisions. That would be the baseline factor that most disposition teams really should take a look at and discuss. How many concepts of those represented on the two opposing teams are you operating under?

DR. CHRIST

Drs. Grunebaum and Goodrich have stirred a lot of interest by not only presenting these perspectives of family therapy, but also the several different ways by which family therapy can be introduced and how each way presents certain problems.

DR. GOODRICH

It is clear from this discussion about how best to go about both doing things and thinking about things that strong loyalties and identifications are being revealed. Perhaps we should see this as simply an expression of the state of our field. In all modesty, psychiatry began to be a real field in the very late 40s, after World War II. It really was not much of a field, academically speaking, until after 1945. Psychiatric research began to grow in the early 1950s throughout the country. Currently, psychiatry is still struggling for a clinical frame of reference and toward some of our very basic operating modalities.

Henry Grunebaum stated that some heads of departments will want to limit the therapeutic approaches or philosophies to one or two or three that are clearly established. In contrast, there are chairmen and directors of services who will be more comfortable with an open-ended organizational structure, perhaps with an internally rivalrous, exciting juxtaposition of many different points of view and different ways of doing things. My own bias to resolve the differences as to the applicability of an analytic approach or brief therapy individual approach or group therapy approach or family approach, or where we have differences among us in conceptual orientations, that the resolution of this is going to be sometimes through confrontations of those who are adherents to different positions. More likely, the resolution will be by individuals who can identify with both sides of the fence. I feel that the best teacher of child psychiatry is one who has had a lot of training in individual therapy and in family therapy, and from that perspective, is better able to make the judgements than if all the experiences have been in one or the other. I am asking for trouble, but that is how I feel.

THINKING LIKE A FAMILY THERAPIST

Henry Grunebaum, M.D. and Richard Chasin, M.D.

Harvard Medical School

Cambridge, Massachusetts

INTRODUCTION

This paper will deal with two interrelated subjects; first, the nature of the family therapy training program we have developed in response to the setting in which we work; and second, the theoretical framework which is the cornerstone of our training program. Family therapy training at the Cambridge Hospital exists in what may be thought of as an educational marketplace of ideas and techniques, and in an institution mandated to care for any and all patients who require service. These two forces have caused us to emphasize theory rather than technique in our training program.

THE TRAINING PROGRAM

Let us now turn first to the characteristics of our setting and the training program which has evolved. The Cambridge Hospital

Dr. Henry Grunebaum is Director, Group and Family Psychotherapy Training, Department of Psychiatry, Cambridge Hospital, Cambridge, Massachusetts and Associate Clinical Professor of Psychiatry, Harvard Medical School.

Dr. Richard Chasin is Assistant Clinical Professor of Psychiatry, Boston University School of Medicine, and Harvard Medical School. He is on the Faculty of the Family Institute, Cambridge, Massachusetts.

is a community mental health center responsible for an urban catchment area where there are significant private resources available
to those who can afford them. We are responsible for teaching
family therapy to psychiatric residents and other mental health
professionals in a training program which begins with an inpatient
year, goes on to a second year in the outpatient department and
includes some general hospital, child psychiatry, and neighborhood
health center experience. Residents then can elect to continue
for an additional specialization in either adult work or in two
years of child psychiatry training. The main thrust of the training
program is psychoanalytic. However, we operate in what may be
thought of as a marketplace of ideas, for along with a predominantly psychoanalytic emphasis, there is significant training
in community psychiatry, psychopharmacology, and biological
psychiatry. In this marketplace, family therapy is merely one
of a number of competing therapies and theories. We do not have
control over the training program, rather we have some influence
on it, but have to compete with others for both the time of the
residents and for resources with which to hire personnel. We
suspect that this situation is the usual one which prevails in
most training centers.

What teaching in community mental health centers demands is
that we must train residents and other professionals to work with
the patients and families who actually come to the center. These
clients often are economically, socially, and educationally disadvantaged, and many are recent immigrants. They tend to be more
disturbed than patients seeking treatment in the private sector.
Frequently, the children are school troublemakers, from fractured
homes and with disinterested or unavailable families. We
cannot approach patients with a "take our treatment or go elsewhere
attitude" since we are the "elsewhere" to which they must go.
The therapeutic alliance with such families is often fragile and
we must work with sensitivity. This means that treatment methods
must be flexible enough to fit each family's needs, not our own
needs. Often, we envy those family therapists who direct their
own training programs either because they run a community facility
their way or because they work in an institution where family
therapy is the prevailing ideology. However, we believe in the
long run that the competition of ideas, the need for breadth of
perspective, and the many encounters with colleagues who are both
supportive and challenging are more useful, more realistic, and
more fun.

In the setting of competing ideas, we must present family
therapy in a way which makes it interesting to the residents who
do not come to us seeking only to learn family therapy. Rather,
the resident wants to learn psychiatry and correctly views family
therapy as merely one aspect of the field. We attempt to convey

a broad theoretical foundation for thinking about families. We
do not expect a resident, most of whose training is directed
towards listening and occasional interpretation as major tools,
will be comfortable immediately in directing family discussions
and prescribing a task to a family. It is our experience that
residents take approximately one year to learn that one can navigate
safely through an interview with a whole family and even learn
something from it. This goal is achieved partly by demonstrating
interviewing the families of ward patients. In the second year,
we teach a seminar on interpersonal psychiatry, 18 hours of which
are devoted to family therapy. We find it is some months into
the second year before the residents see how the individual
patients with whom they are working can be understood in terms of
their family context. However, it takes even more time before
they begin to work with family units. Only toward the end of the
second year, when the residents grow frustrated by the effort of
confining their work to talk and empathy, is it possible to
interest them in giving families tasks to undertake.

When they begin child psychiatry, the situation is somewhat
different. Here again, however, the effects of the structure of
the institutions where we work influences what it is possible to
accomplish. Usually parents tend to be seen by social workers, and
children by residents. This system mitigates against family
units being seen as a whole. However, in the part of the catchment
area that is most economically deprived, and where the clinic is
less well-staffed, it is more common for families to be seen by
one person. The training of child psychiatry fellows in family
therapy is conducted in much the same way as in previous years.
They participate in seminars, observe live interviews, interview
families themselves both alone and with co-therapists, and receive
supervision. Infrequently, interviews are done behind a one-way
mirror since this educational device is not readily available--nor
is a videotape machine.

In both child and adult psychiatry, the trainees are exposed
to a wide variety of therapeutic modalities and theories. What
we are trying to teach is that every patient and every family must
be conceptualized as a family whether or not they are treated
as a unit. We would agree with Murray Bowen who says "think
family." This lesson is more important to learn than the detailed
skills of conjoint interviewing. Finally, we are impressed that
over the three or four years following completion of training, the
junior staff becomes increasingly interested in work with families
and couples and seek us out for consultation and case discussion.

A THEORY OF FAMILY THERAPY

While a part of the difficulty in becoming a family therapist

has to do with the newness and discomfort involved in work with
multiperson units, we believe a more significant difficulty arises
from the lack of clarity about what data one should observe and
how one should attempt to influence the family. Central to our
thinking is the belief that there are three basic ways of looking
at families, or for that matter individuals, and that these perspectives are all equally and simultaneously valid.[1]

All concepts about family functioning and all methods of
analyzing family pathology observe and evaluate the family from
at least one of three perspectives: (1) the historical perspective
where the evaluation is an effort to learn about the past origins
of the family predicament; (2) interactional perspective, where
the evaluation attempts to observe recurrent family interactions
and to deduce underlying rules and structures; and, (3) the
existential perspective where the evaluation attempts to
apprehend the subjective quality of an individual's experience
within the family.

A key element in our thinking is that all interventions are
based on one or more of three different treatment approaches,
each of which corresponds to a major way in which people learn.
They are: (1) the understanding approach, where the intervention
by explaining increases the families' knowledge about its past
and current functioning and experience. This approach is based
on cognitive learning. (2) the transformation approach, where
the intervention is designed to change family interaction in some
significant way, often by the assignment of tasks--this approach

---

[1]The closest similar effort to the one we will attempt is that by
Scheflen (1978), in his clearly thought out yet charming paper;
"Susan Smiled: On Explanation in Family Therapy." Scheflen states
"The Contemporary pschotherapist is exposed to a variety of conceptual models and paradigms. These are usually presented as
opposing truths in different doctoral schools, but actually they
are all valid from one point of view or another. And accordingly,
they are all tactically useful at some point or another" (p. 7).
He then delineates that Susan's smile can be considered variously
as "an expression, a response, a stimulus, a patterned response,
a meta response, and finally as an intrapersonal expression.
Clearly, Scheflen believes that each of these explanations of
Susan's smile, and what relation or lack of relation the smile had
to what preceded and followed it, are all equally potentially
explanatory and tactically useful. We will approach the same
problem from a somewhat different standpoint, which we hope
will also help to clarify the nature of explanation in work with
families.

is based on learning by behavioral conditioning; and (3) the identification approach, where the intervention is designed to create new models for behavior often by the therapists' example, but sometimes through the introduction of significant figures from the past such as parents so that old identifications may be modified--this approach is based on learning through imitation and identification.

We are not here emphasizing that each member of the family has his or her own viewpoint about the family and that these are all valid and important, although that is true. Nor are we emphasizing that the therapist's own view of the family is yet another perspective, neither more or less valid than that of anyone else. Rather, we are highlighting that there are three different ways of viewing any given happening in a family.

At this point, it is useful to say something about the difference between family therapy and family thinking, because it is the latter in which we are primarily interested. Family therapy has been viewed by outsiders and beginners as a form of therapy in which it is useful, perhaps even necessary, for all members of the designated patient's immediate family to be seen simultaneously by one or more therapists in the same room and at the same time. In point of fact, we are impressed from an informal survey of our colleagues that this mode of work tends to occur rather infrequently, no more than perhaps 5 - 15 percent of the therapy hours of active family therapists. More commonly, family therapists are seeing couples, and more often they are working with individuals. Clearly, it is not the number of people present that determines whether or not family therapy is occurring, it is the approach towards the work that makes the difference. In fact, some inexperienced therapists see families conjointly and yet treat them as a collection of individuals.

We, therefore, believe that the distinctive contributions of family therapy are theoretical rather than technical. It is these theoretical concepts that the student needs most to learn. Once the theory is grasped, the student can start to develop comfort interviewing the traditional family, a wide variety of families such as several children and two parents; the more common and less discussed ones such as the parents of a psychotic young adult; the divorced sets of parents of a disturbed child; the grown child of a psychotic older person; the single parent with a delinquent child; and, the psychotic mother and her infant. We attempt to give our students the necessary theoretical framework and the basic skills to deal with the problems they actually encounter.

THE THREE PERSPECTIVES FOR EVALUATION

In the evaluation of families, there are three basic questions a family therapist can ask of, and about, a family: (1) How have things come to be this way? (2) What is going on now? (3) What is it like to be in this family now? The first question is an historic inquiry in which one is interested in the story of the family, how it got to be where it is, what have been its traditions and secrets, its expectations and hopes, its tragedies and joys. The second question focuses attention on family interaction. It views the family as a system which can be observed from the outside. One asks: "What makes things happen the way they are now?" One is likely to notice that the family is acting as though certain interactions had a repetitive and inevitable quality. The third question concerns itself with the experience of each member of the family and of the therapist as he/she sits with the family and becomes involved with them and their experience. One is interested in what it feels like to be a member of this family. We are interested in the family climate. Some families are happy, others joyless, and still others are both.

A good automobile mechanic would understand our three per-spectives. When you bring your car into the repair shop, he/she might ask about history: "What on earth happened to this thing?" Or, he/she might be convinced by you that really nothing has happened to it that you know of, but he may identify some structural damage or some faulty interaction among the parts. Or, failing to do these he might say: "I'd like to road test it. I want to find out what it's like to drive this car." A chess board is another analogy. An historical perspective question might be, "How did this position develop?" An interactional question is: "However it developed, can we have a mate in three?" The existential question is: "What would it be like to be a pawn that is one box away from becoming a queen with the opposite queen and two castles bearing down on it?"

1. The historical perspective. Let us now turn to a discussion of the historical perspective in family therapy. We view this perspective as an effort to understand family relation-ships and transactions that are the precipitates of the family's history. This perspective is well illustrated by Ivan Borz-ormeny-Nagy and Geraldine Spark in their book Invisible Loyalties (1973) which is adumbrated and obscure but, nonetheless, makes a tremendous emotional impression on the reader.

The central theme is that families are intensely attached units which pass on traditions to the next generation even if the tradition paradoxically is one of detachment, disinterest, and disengagement. The tradition of families is not simply a matter

of ethnicity, race, creed, and culture, or even the unique cultures
of families but involves a moral dimension of debits and credits
in a ledger of justice which each member keeps. Such debits and
credits are not simply paid by those who owe them to those to
whom they are owed, but rather that they are transferred to other
generations. People who have been well-treated by their parents
may feel they owe their children the same, while those who have
been deprived by their parents may deprive their own children and
indeed expect their children to nurture them. This, Nagy and
Spark (1973) call "the parentification of a child."[2]

In treatment, one can use loyalty explanations as they are
well accepted by families. Thus, we can point out that by not
putting down roots, the child of parents who have survived the
Holocaust is loyal to their uprooted experience. Such interpretations give the family a fresh perspective on behaviors,
even those apparently discordant with family norms as being
connected to a family life rather than an expression of some in-
comprehensible evil in a child. A further reason why we believe
that "loyalty explanations" are so well accepted is that "loyalty"
is part of the ongoing existential experience of each member of
the family striking a resonance with deeply felt emotional ties.

Certainly, there is a long tradition in family therapy of
history taking beginning with Nathan Ackerman (1959), and going
up to the present. We make note that Minuchin (1974) and
Palazzoli (1977), who work from a structural (interactional) perspective, usually begin a case study with historical material.
For instance, Palazzoli (1978) states in the very first sentence
of a chapter on "The Family of the Anorectic and the Social
Environment," "Our twelve families all shared one major characteristic. They tried to preserve agricultural-patriarchal values,
roles, rules and taboos in an urban-industrial setting" (p. 242).
Thus, misplaced loyalty is a central theme in her work even
though what she stresses is the current family structure (interactional pattern). We cite this example to clarify that therapists
use all three. Later, we will discuss the relationships between
the three perspectives and the three approaches.

2. The interactional perspective. Let us now turn to the
interactional perspective, where the therapist is interested in
observing the family's current interactions and take the position

---

[2]Without any inquiry into history, Minuchin (1974) might call a
"parentified child" a parental child simply by observing the
child playing a parent's role in the current family interaction.

of the uninvolved behavior. Therapists who have pioneered in
the interactional perspective have differed along three major
parameters: first, in the degree to which they pay attention to
fine details (interactional analysis) or the broad sweep of
interaction (study of family structure); second, the scope of
their field of observation (ranging from couples to extended
networks; and, third, the particular behaviors they are most
interested in ranging from characteristics of communication to
the details of sexual activity, to the sequence of family transactions.

Since the interactional perspective is both less familiar and
more complicated to most readers, we will review the work of
several important groups beginning with the observers of communication (who came first historically). There are two principal
contributions to the study of communication: first, the "Double-
Bind" theorists, namely, Bateson, Jackson, Haley, and Weakland
(1971) who were interested primarily in schizophrenia and in
communication pairs, and second, Virginia Satir (1967), who was
interested in healthier families and their communication as it
blocked normal growth and development.

The Palo Alto group (Bateson, Jackson, Haley, and Weakland)
who developed the theory of the double-bind began with an
interest in the study of the theory of logic and, in particular,
the logic of classes. They suggested that a particular form of
miscommunication (which they called the double-bind) occurred
when five requirements were met: (1) there was a strong positive
communication, usually in words; (2) an equally strong negative
injunction, usually nonverbal; (3) the demand for action; (4) no
opportunity to leave the field; and, (5) no metacommunication by
which they meant no discussion of the muddle the individual was
placed in. This, they believed to be characteristic of parents
relating to their schizophrenic offspring. Now, many years after
this very stimulating and much studied theory was first proposed,
we are still not able to reach firm conclusions about its status.
Research does not support the view that the double-bind is truly
characteristic of the parents of schizophrenics; indeed, it is
not even clear if the theory is testable. It should be noted
that the theory is an "interactional" theory in the sense that
interaction implies the influence of parents on the child, but
does not take a fully interactional point of view, namely, that
each is influenced by the other. Thus, the theory is a one-way
theory, the parents do it to the child. In addition, it is not
clear which postulates are of most importance. For instance, no
escape from the family may well be pathogenic in and of itself.
Finally, it is a theory of communicating dyads, not triads or
more. Nonetheless, it has been enormously influential and has
focused much attention on family communication and miscommunication and on levels of communicating and miscommunicating.

Virginia Satir (1967), is interested in families facing more normal developmental crisis and in helping people to "level" with each other, and the characteristic ways they do and fail to do so. She described four modes of miscommunicating which appear as positions individuals characteristically assume during inter-action sequences. She calls these modes survivor positions. People use them when they find themselves in situations of stress or where self-esteem is at stake. They are: (1) the placating stance " anything you want," "you first" (this stance attempts to avoid attack); (2) the blaming stance, attacking the other to gain a feeling of safety and strength; (3) the computer stance, a cold and logical position designed to avoid having one's feelings involved in the outcome; and (4) the irrelevance stance, avoid the issue by diversions and distracting. Satir, looks at each communication during an interaction characterizing it as levelling (normal) communication or as one of the four types of dysfunctional communication stances.

Before going on to discuss more recent contributors to the interactional perspective, it may be helpful to say a little about the present usefulness of communication as the behavior to be observed. It is our impression that while research on communication such as that of Wynne and Singer (1965) on "trans-actional thought disorder," and Mishler and Waxler (1968), par-ticularly with schizophrenics has been of great interest, the clinical utility of concentrating on communication has not been great. It may be of help to families to note unclear communica-tions, but it is difficult for families to change their styles of communicating. More effective has been the effort to help members of families talk to the particular person they wish to communicate with; in other words, to focus on targets of messages. Probably, therapists mistakenly believe that patients should resemble them and thus be verbal and interested in talk. However, there is little evidence to support the view that talkative as opposed to laconic couples are better adjusted or that frequency of communications rated as positive as opposed to negative are reflected in marital happiness.

More recently, David Kantor (1975) has been interested in studying the positions each family takes by taping families as they go about their daily lives. He defines our psychopolitical positions: "initiators, opposers, followers, and bystanders." An individual may take a different position depending on what the goal, or as Kantor (1975) says, "the target" of the communication is. He believes there are three main goals of family interaction; "affect, power, and meaning." He maintains that there is nothing inherently pathological about the positions an individual assumes as long as he/she can change when necessary and not get stuck. This reminds one of the conclusion of Mishler and Waxler (1965) that healthy families' communications are marked by inter-

ruptions and humor, while only pathological familes speak in
sequence.

Probably the most important contribution to the interactional
perspective has been made by Bowen (1978) and Minuchin (1974)
whose works are impossible to summarize easily. Both have shown
interest in failures of individuals to become independent from
their families of origin: failures which Bowen might call being
undifferentiated and Minuchin might call being enmeshed. Both
have been interested in stable coalitions in families usually
between one parent and a child which renders the other parent
ineffective and, indeed, the parental coalition ineffective.
Here, it is worth noting that it was Lidz (1965) who first drew
attention to the importance of boundaries between parents and
children and between the sexes in families. Both Bowen and
Minuchin attempt to restructure the family to alter the distribu-
tion of power, returning it to the parents and removing the child
as the symptom bearer for difficulties in the husband-wife relationship. Bowen usually does this by working with the healthiest
members of the family and attempts to "detriangulate" the
symptomatic member while Minuchin works with the whole family and
forces a reallocation of control to the parents.

While the structural perspective of Bowen and Minuchin is
often focused on triangles which they discern by observing recurrent interaction sequence in families, both have evolved
concepts to explain the over-involvement of family members with
one another and their inabilities to individuate. Enmeshment
and undifferentiation sound very much like perversions of
loyalty and are reminiscent of the work of Nagy and Spark (1973).
If one reads the case histories presented, particularly by
Minuchin (1974), one often has the feeling that the family is
enmeshed because the parents espouse a tradition of loyalty
appropriate in the past but dysfunctional in the present.

This brief overview of the interactional perspective has
highlighted the contributions of Satir (1967) and Bateson, et al
(1956), who have emphasized communicative behavior and Minuchin
(1974), and Bowen (1978) who have studied affiliation and power
structures in families. We believe that these two areas have
received the greatest attention and have greatly influenced family
therapists. However, it is important to take note of the fact
that arising out of the traditions of behavior therapy, workers
such as Patterson (1975), Weiss (1976), Lieberman (1976), and
Jacobson (1976), have begun to look at family interaction with
an eye towards altering maladaptive interaction with changes in
conditioning and reenforcement. These approaches are better
known to behavior therapists than to family therapists. In the
years to come, there will likely be a rapprochment between family
and behavior therapists (Birk /1974/ is a pioneer in this area),

since the latter are finding that an individual's family is likely
to be the most powerful reenforcers of his/her behavior, and
detailed attention to the behaviors which can be observed in
families is of growing interest to family therapists. It is
important to note that central to the interactional perspective
is the idea that the therapist is an observer of the family.
He/she must attempt to remain outside the family, see what goes
on among family members, and intervene to change behavior usually
by prescribing a different behavior or task for the family to
undertake.

3. <u>The existential perspective</u>. This perspective takes the
position that it is vital for the therapist to become aware of
and take into account the ongoing experience of each member of the
family as well as his/her own experience as an outsider entering
the family. More than anything else, it requires empathy, a
willingness to identify with the feelings and views of each member
of the family. The therapist must get inside the family.
Obviously, there will be those individuals and families who are
easy to identify with and those who are more difficult. Nonetheless, we do not believe that in the long run, family therapy
can be successful unless each person present feels understood.
We are aware that many family therapists make a conscious effort
to ally themselves with each member of the family, and this is
useful, if not necessary. However, the effort to ally is
different from the effort to empathize with another human being.
The former has a specific therapeutic objective in mind, the
latter none other than the effort to respect another person by
attempting to experience their life as they do. We believe it is
useful to clarify the differences between this perspective and the
two preceding ones. We are impressed that it is possible to
teach students how to take historical and interactional perspectives, but it is far more difficult to help them empathize with
all of the members. This is particularly true of younger trainees
who are still attempting to individuate and to come to terms with
their own parents and families of origin.

Reading the family therapy literature leads us to believe
that while most experienced family therapists believe that
empathy with the family is important (Haley, 1976, is perhaps an
exception), it is not specifically described as a separate
perspective but simply as part of the task of the therapist. This
is different from schools of individual therapy where the existential therapists, as Havens has described in "Approaches to
the Mind" (1973), make an effort, however difficult it may be,
to remain in an empathic bond which is essential to the therapy.
Nonetheless, certain family therapists have described findings
which require the therapist to experience the family as though he
were a member of it (Fogarty, 1976) or by helping family members
appraise their emotional responses within the family.

Bowen has described the concept of differentiation of the self with the family.   He believes that any individual can be placed on the dimension of differentiation or lack of differentiation which measures the ability to experience and acknowledge one's own feelings while remaining a member of one's family.   In order for an individual to gauge his/her level of differentiation, Bowen (1978) may say the following: "If you can go to your family of origin and talk with each member of the family for about twenty minutes, during which time you do not talk about the weather or other people, but just talk about yourself and your feelings and thoughts about the other person, and you can do that and be reasonable, rather than only emotionally reactive, and not get sucked in, then you are a fully differentiated person. However, if in talking with the members of your family, you feel bound in, overreactive, drawn into old fights, and talking to the other person the way that you used to, to that extent you are not yet differentiated." Clearly, it is how one feels in one's family that makes the difference for Bowen.

In Bowen's terms no one is fully differentiated. Where we would differ from Bowen is that we do not believe that full differentiation is even desirable, for being a member of a family is to have a sense of rootedness and of history, that old patterns remain alive even though altered or diminished in silence, and that old feelings are still present even though they are shadows and memories rather than the current reality. However, in terms of the existential perspective, the sense of oneself as a separate person that Bowen has delineated is clearly a key element.

Fogarty (1976) has also been interested in the concept of self-differentiation. However, he asks the question: What is it that makes differentiation so difficult? His answer is that in order to differentiate, one must confront one's essential aloneness in the world and the feelings of emptiness that arise if one gives up the hope that others can alleviate this feeling. Fogarty believes that in order to help a patient to differentiate, the therapist must deal with the depression that arises inevitably as a consequence of the loss of using others to solve problems which are one's own. Considering Bowen's work, one is led naturally to the question of what interferes with the differentiation. Here we find a link between family systems and individual psychodynamics using the concept of projective identification as a bridge. What prevents differentiation is that one is caught up by one's tendency to use one's significant others to complete oneself, that one is not complete alone—to supply missing aspects of the self. One can do this by projecting attributes on to another or receiving attributes from another. In all these operations, aspects of the self are disowned, split off, and projected onto the other person, who is then identified within a close relationship and experienced

as possessing or containing these attributes. Finally, as Laing
(1971) has emphasized, the other person is pressured to comply
with the projections and act in accordance with the disowned parts
of the self. Indeed, they are either molded if they are a child,
or are selected if they are a spouse to fit with the disowned parts
of the self so that they come to act a familiar and necessary
part in order to make the self feel complete and full.

     Of all the family therapists, it is Nagy and Spark (1973) who
have most clearly contributed to the historical perspective. They
have described the importance of justice, accountability, and fair-
ness within families. Members may feel they have been treated
unjustly by parents and they are owed a debt, a debt which children
or spouse may be asked to pay but which is really owed by the
parents. The sense that one is owed something or that one owes
something to others is clearly an essential inner experience, unique
and powerful. It links one inextricably with others and prevents
one's differentiation. One does not simply have the feeling which
Bowen describes that one is still caught up in old patterns and
cannot be oneself, but rather the deeper feeling that one cannot
be oneself and does not want to until old accounts are paid and
the ledger of justice is balanced.

THREE TREATMENT APPRAOCHES

     Let us now turn to the three approaches to treatment. In an
approach based on Understanding, the therapist interprets past
influences and illuminates current patterns in order to enrich the
family's knowledge of the origin and nature of its present
predicament. In an approach based on Transformation, the therapist
strategically directs the family in order to modify and correct
its dysfunctional transactions, sequences and structure. In an
approach based on Identification, the living model of the therapist
and the active involvement of older family members promote new
identifications and relaxes the grip of destructive introjects and
pointless loyalties among family members. We recognize that the
therapy of any particular family inevitably involves a blend of
these approaches. Nonetheless, we believe it is useful for us to
examine each approach separately in order to organize intelligently
the complex array of techniques used in family therapy.

     One reason for selecting the categories of understanding,
transformation, and identification, is that each of these approaches
corresponds to each of the three ways children learn and change.
Parents teach their children by their increasing knowldge (understanding), by modifying their behavior patterns (transformation),
and by setting an example (identification).

     In order to be effective, the techniques used in each of the approaches ought to conform to the principles that underly the corresponding mode of learning. Therefore, in an approach based on understanding, the therapist would do well to be a fascinating and lucid teacher. In an approach based on transformation, the therapist needs to pay vigilant attention to motivation, cooperation and contingencies of reward and punishment. In an approach based on identification, the therapist must be ready to offer himself or herself for intimate and intense interaction with the family.

In a fascinating paper, Loevinger (1971), suggests the reason that parents fail all too often relates to the three modes of learning. She points out that the child is always able to view the tactic used by the parent according to a different theory of learning than the one the parent thought he/she was using. Thus, spanking a child for hitting intended to be aversion, but can be experienced as an opportunity for imitation or identification and lead to more hitting. Similarly, an effort at explanation and understanding by a parent can be experienced either as too mild or too severe a behavioral reinforcer, with the child feeling either, "I got away with it that time," or "Another dreadful lecture by Mom or Dad!"

We are impressed that patients are not essentially different from children or anyone else who is able to learn or change. We are all free, and perhaps, in fact our freedom resides in the ability to view and react to efforts to influence us by thinking about them differently at different times. Patients and individuals seeking assistance with problems will experience the therapist in terms of all modes of learning. The therapist cannot help but be simultaneously a source of understanding, a sharer of frustration, and finally a model.

Problems in therapy can often be explained when the therapist does not appreciate the three ways he/she influences the patient. Many failures of therapy we believe have been due to too narrow an approach to how people learn and change. For instance, Applebaum (1972) has discussed in a paper on psychoanalysis that being in analysis can be a pleasant experience, so pleasant in fact, that the patient may seek to avoid changing in order to avoid losing this rare human opportunity. On the other hand, the therapist may dispassionately aid the family in understanding the source and nature of its frozen intellectualization, but the family may learn only to identify with additional patterns of detachment modeled by their cool and distant therapist. Behavioral therapists similarly have increasingly found it necessary to explain why they are engaged in the particular behavior tactics they are employing and at times even to explore some of the patient's feelings about their therapist.

1. The understanding approach (Explaining). Techniques

used in the understanding approach all have the object of helping the family see what the therapist sees from each of the three evaluation perspectives. Thus, the total of such techniques may be to help the family grasp the way its behavior results from the flow of historical forces; it might be to help them be aware of the exact way their interactive sequences work to frustrate each other's needs; it might help them to be aware of their own inner experience and empathize with the subjective life of other family members.

Family therapists have been enormously inventive in developing techniques for improving family self-awareness from all three perspectives. Diaries, photo albums, taped interviews with old family friends and relatives, even dramatic improvisations of past events have all been used to shed light on family history. In the effort to teach families about the nature of their interactions and structure, family therapists have shown families videotape playbacks of spontaneous family discussions as well as playbacks of themselves performing standardized family tasks. Family sculpting, drawing pictures of the family, and role playing have all been employed to help the family be aware of the quality of experience each member has inside the family.

2. The transformation approach (Shaping). The second category of approaches is called transformation. The techniques encompassed by this approach all share the characteristic of being centered about activities directed or induced by the therapist and performed by one or more family members. These activities are designed to improve the nature of family interactions even if the activity does not increase the family's understanding of itself.

This definition pulls into one category techniques that originate in a wide variety of schools of psychotherapy. It includes techniques from behavior modification, strategic psychotherapy, structural family therapy, communication focused family therapy, Bowenian therapy, Gestalt therapy, and psychodrama.

In creating this conglomerate of techniques, we do not intend to erase the important differences that exist in the theories and practices of the therapies from which they are derived; rather, we draw attention to their common elements. They involve tasks prescribed by therapists often with no explanation. Since tasks may meet with considerable family resistance, some practitioners use subtle methods for obtaining client compliance such as those practiced by hypnotists like Milton Erikson (1973).

In prescribing tasks, the therapist may use straightforward directives or strategic directives. A straightforward directive often prescribes a task that obviously might directly benefit the family situation.

Most directives are straightforward. They are usually aimed
at small items of interaction as opposed to sequences or structure.
For example, a family member may be instructed to improve the
content of his communications:

> Therapist: "John, when you are ready, tell Mary
>   exactly how you feel."

Or, he may be instructed to alter the style and language of his
communications:

> Therapist: "John when talking about feelings, try
>   to start sentences with the word "I."
>   Avoid telling Mary how <u>she</u> feels. If
>   you want to know how she feels, <u>ask</u> her."

Sometimes, straightforward directives are pointed at sequences:

> Therapist: "John and Mary, I want you both to
>   listen carefully to Peggy. Whenever
>   she complains, I want you to thank her.
>   Peggy, see if you can complain once in
>   this meeting, but don't do it unless it
>   feels safe."

Finally, directives may deal with structure:

> Therapist: "John, I think that your wife and
>   daughter have some things to talk
>   over woman-to-woman. Let's permit
>   them to talk privately. Come here
>   and tell me about this collection
>   of old photos you've started. (The
>   therapist is trying to alter a
>   structure that has a father/daughter
>   coalition.)

All of the above directives were straightforward as opposed to
strategic directives which involve tasks that may not be beneficial in themselves, but which are designed to lead indirectly
to beneficial changes in family interactions and structure. For
example, a couple who were having no sexual life were instructed
to prepare a sumptuous dinner together. That activity led by
analogy to other types of combined pleasure.

Paradoxical instructions are strategic. If a defiant boy who
fights continually with his sister is told to have ten fights
with her in the following week, he might have only five. By
prescribing the symptom it loses its systems function. Fighting

is no longer defiant. The directive produces an effect anticipated
by the therapist but not by the family.

3. Identification (Exemplifying). In all family therapy,
clients form new identifications and modify old ones through
imitation of, or identification with, the person of the therapist.
In stranger group therapy, such changes in identification occur
not only in relationship with the therapist, but with the other
clients as well. In family therapy, family members may be even
more powerful in affecting identification than are therapists
or other members of a stranger group.

Thus, the potential for changes in identification may be at
its greatest when one shares the therapy with one's parents, the
most critical source of one's original key identifications. It
is tempting to believe that during interaction with our parents,
our old identifications are still malleable--even long after
childhood has past.

Plausible explanation of this phenomenon relates to family
loyalties. Inextricably woven into the fabric of our identifications
is our sense of what we are owed and what we owe others. Much of
this inner sense of expectation and obligation comes directly
from the behavior and statements of our parents. If our parents
originally helped to establish our obligations, can they not also
release us from them and thus help us modify this decisive aspect
of our identifications?

In conclusion and by way of summing, we will discuss the
relationship between the three perspectives, the three approaches
and the stance of the therapist. As we have suggested, it is both
natural and indeed usual for the information gathered through
each perspective to be employed by using a particular approach;
it is usual but it is not necessary or even always optimal. Thus,
often a therapist gathers history and grasps its importance on the
current situation, it seems natural for most therapists to use an
understanding approach to treatment; that is, for the therapist to
help the family learn about itself by using clarification and interpretation. Similarly, it is natural for most therapists who study
maladaptive interactive patterns and structures to try to use
transformation techniques designed to improve family conduct and
structures. Finally, therapists who study the subjective experience
of each family member (how they are in the world), often use
themselves and older family members as a source for shifting
identities. Thus, the following links appear natural: historical
perspective with understanding approach, interactional perspective
with transformation approach, experiential perspective with
identification approach. However, all possible links between
perspective and approach occur. After gathering data principally

from an historical perspective, the therapist may decide to use
mainly transformational techniques.

The different perspective approaches lead to quite different
stances in terms of the distance and objectivity of the therapist
and the use of his/her authority. Therapists who use understanding
will tend to be somewhat distant so that they may observe without
becoming overly involved. They will attempt to be supportive but
not too emotional; and they will state their understanding of
dynamics, either individual or familial, in an authoritative way,
but without the expectation that action should follow understanding
immediately, or even necessarily. On the other hand, therapists
who observe interaction and deduce structure will tend to keep
their observations more to themselves, since understanding is not
necessary for change. Rather, they will devise tasks to transform
family behavior. They will keep enough distance both to observe
the family objectively and to maintain the requisite position of
authority. Indeed, if the task appears to be peculiar, if not
ridiculous, the therapist may need to be authoritative if not
authoritarian. Finally, the therapist using the identification
approach will attempt to minimize the distance betwen himself/
herself and the family. Objectivity is a distancing maneuver, for
a therapist cannot remain an outside observer and at the same time
experience the plight of the family empathically. In the effort
to foster identifications with him/her, the therapist may share
with the family his/her own feelings and experiences. Events
of an experiential nature cannot be planned; rather they must
arise naturally--it is true that the soil in which they can occur
can be prepared. The family must feel safe, cared for, and
understood both as a group and as individuals.

No matter what the approach, the attitude of the therapist's
behavior must reflect concern for the family and the intention
to be beneficial. This attitude is particularly important for
therapists who prescribe difficult or uncomprehensible tasks.
Their stance may be distant, but they must show the commitment
to help. Since no therapist can be all things to all families,
all trainees and therapists need to learn their own favored
stances and most congenial approaches. They must also be aware
that some families will be hard for them to care about. This
awareness should guide case selection and should raise questions
about matters to be resolved between the therapist and his/her
own family.

Different families or the same family at different times in
their lives, or in the course of therapy, will respond differ-
entially to the stance of the therapist. We do not believe that
there is one therapy for all patients, or that any given therapist
can be all things to all families. Rather, we think that

therapists should have some sense of the range of possibilities open to them--to explore in depth or in breadth as their predilections and lives take them.

REFERENCES

Ackerman, N. Emotional impact of in-laws and relatives. In: Samuel Liebman (Ed.), Emotional Forces in the Family, Philadelphia:Lippincott, 1959.

Applebaum, A. A critical re-examination of the concept "Motivation for change" in psychoanalytic treatment. International Journal of Psychoanalysis, 53:51-59, 1972.

Bateson, G., Jackson, D., Haley, J., and Weakland, J. Toward a theory of schizophrenia. In: J. Howells (Ed.) Theory and Practice of Family Psychiatry, New York: Brunner/Mazel, 1971, pp. 745-764.

Birk, L. and Brinkley-Birk, A. Psychoanalysis and behavior therapy, American Journal of Psychiatry, 131:5, pp. 499-510, May, 1974.

Boszormeny-Nagy, I. and Spark, G. M. Invisible Loyalties. Cambridge: Harvard University Press, 1973.

Bowen, M. Family Therapy in Clinical Practice. New York: Jason Aronson, 1978.

Fogarty, T. On Emptiness and Closeness, Part I and Part II. Center for Family Learning, New Rochelle, New York, 1976.

Haley, J. Problem Solving Therapy. San Francisco:Jossey Bass, 1976.

Havens, L. Approaches to the Mind: Movement of the Psychiatric Schools from Sects Toward Science. Boston:Little Brown, 1973.

Jacobson, N. S. and Martin, B. Behavioral marriage therapy: current status. Psychological Bulletin, 85:540-556, 1976.

Kantor, D. Inside the Family. San Francisco:Jossey Bass, 1975.

Laing, R. D. Sanity, Madness and the Family. New York:Basic Books, 1971.

Lidz, T., Fleck, S., and Cornelison, A. Schizophrenia and the Family. New York:International Universities Press, 1965.

Liberman, R. P., Levine, J., Wheeler, E., Sanchers, N., and Wallace, C. Experimental evaluation of marital group therapy: Behavioral versus Interaction, Insight, Comments. Acta. Psychiatry Scandiv., 1976

Loevinger, J. Patterns of parenthood as theories of learning. In: A. Skolnick and H. H. Skolnick (Eds.) Family in Transition, Boston:Little Brown, 1971, pp. 342-346.

Minuchin, S. Families and Family Therapy. Cambridge:Harvard University Press, 1974.

Mishler, E. and Waxler, N. Interaction in Families. New York: Wiley, 1968.

Mishler, E. and Waxler, N. Family interaction process and schizophrenia: A review of current theories. Reprinted from Merrill-Palmer Quarterly:Behavior and Development Series, 1965, pp. 269-315.

Palazzoli, M. S., Boscolo, L., Cecchin, C. F., and Prata, G.
    Family rituals: A powerful tool in family therapy. Family
    Process, 16:445-453, 1977.
Patterson, G. R., Weiss, R. L., Hop, H. Training of marital skills.
    In: H. Leitenberg (Ed.) Handbook of Behavior Modification
    and Behavior Therapy. New York:Prentice Hall, 1976.
Satir, V. Conjoint Family Therapy. Palo Alto: Science and
    Behavior Books, 1967.
Scheflen, A. E. Susan smiled: On explanation in family therapy.
    Family Process, March, 1978, 17:59-68.
Weiss, R. L. and Margolis, G. Marital conflict and accord. In:
    A. R. Ciminero, H. D. Calhoun, and H. E. Adams (Eds.)
    Handbook for Behavioral Assessment. New York:Wiley, 1976.
Wynne, L. and Singer, M. Thought disorder and family relationships
    of schizophrenics. Archives of General Psychiatry, 12:
    187-212 III and IV, 1965.

THE THEORETICAL PERSPECTIVE IN TEACHING FAMILY THERAPY: DISCUSSION

OF DR. GRUNEBAUM'S AND DR. CHASIN'S PAPER

Charles A. Malone, M.D.

Case Western Reserve University

Cleveland, Ohio

It is a pleasure to have the opportunity to begin the discussion
of Dr. Grunebaum's and Dr. Chasin's stimulating if, at times,
difficult to follow, paper. While the paper does not focus
mainly on curriculum design, or child psychiatry training per se,
it clearly articulates a way of conceptualizing family therapy
which has many implications for teaching family therapy in relation
to child psychiatry training. Since, in the brief time allotted
to me, it would be impossible to discuss all, or even most, of the
interesting issues raised by this paper, I will confine my comments
to several areas which have particular significance for me.

Dr. Grunebaum and Dr. Chasin correctly point out that there
are different theoretical perspectives for viewing any given
happening in a family, each with its own actual or potential
validity as a means of understanding pathological family patterns
and as a basis for therapeutic interventions. While these different
perspectives are reflected in the work of major contributors to the
field of family therapy, the authors wisely avoid treating the
variety of conceptual models of family therapy as opposing truths.
Instead they attempt to provide their residents with the necessary
theoretical framework to deal with the clinical problems they
actually encounter. Believing that it is the approach to clinical
work rather than the number of people seen or the format used
which determines whether family therapy is occurring or not,
Dr. Grunebaum and Dr. Chasin attempt to teach their residents how
to "think family" as Bowen puts it.

Central to the paper and to the authors' teaching is a way of
thinking about families which provides clarity about what data one
should collect and how one should attempt to influence families.

This involves three basic ways of looking at families--the historical perspective, the behavioral-structural perspective, and the exper- iential perspective--and three models of family treatment--the insight-understanding approach, the strategic-behavioral approach, and the emotional experience-modeling approach. They caution, however, that one must avoid the natural and historical tendency to pair perspectives and treatment approaches (e.g., the historical perspective with the insight-understanding treatment approach). Dr. Grunebaum and Dr. Chasin do, however, link the three treatment approaches with the ways that children learn--by widening awareness and deepening understanding, by reinforcement or extinction of behavior, and by imitation and identification.

It seems to me that there are a number of advantages to this teaching method.

1. It avoids polarization between insight oriented treatment and family systems therapy. It seems to me that this is essential in any training program which has, as does the one in which Dr. Grunebaum and Dr. Chasin teach, a strong commitment to teaching residents analytically oriented individual psychotherapy. While they do not mention it, since their conceptual model includes the insight oriented treatment approach, I would imagine that it is critical to the effectiveness of their teaching to translate transactional process and the structural, behavioral or experiential techniques related to it into dynamic intrapsychic terms and vice versa; that it is vital to develop the residents' understanding of the interrelationship between individual psychology and trans- actional family process.

2. The conceptual framework developed by Dr. Grunebaum and Dr. Chasin can reduce resident confusion regarding the proliferation of techniques which has occurred in the field of family therapy. It can assist residents in collecting and organizing data, planning treatment, and choosing among techniques, being clear about the theory of learning being used. Residents are taught to categorize techniques according to therapeutic goals. This appears to be an effective way of reducing cookbook imitations of techniques and increasing the residents' understanding that the multiple clinical approaches which characterize the field of family may not, in fact, represent distinct forms of treatment. The conceptual framework also provides a means of reviewing the work of major contributors to the field, identifying the perspectives employed, and the treatment approaches utilized. Of course, this review must be done with a clear recognition, as the authors acknowledge, that the categories overlap and that family therapists such as Nagy, Bowen, Paul and others do not fit readily into a single perspective or a single treatment approach.

3. The teaching method used by Dr. Grunebaum and Dr. Chasin

fits very well with the "marketplace of ideas" type of residency
in which they operate. While they do not complain about it, I
would imagine that not having control over the training program
presents problems--for example, the splitting of families in
child psychiatry with social workers seeing the parents and
residents seeing the child. On the contrary, they appear to welcome
the competition for the residents' interest involved in their
training program and set realistic goals regarding what residents
can be expected to learn at each year level. On the other hand,
their model places high demands on the residents' ability to
integrate theory with practice and this presents a problem as well
as a paradox which I will comment on later. Their conceptual
model can be taught in a weekly family therapy seminar and
reinforced through supervision around clinical assignments.
Interestingly, they do not expect their residents to become family
therapists but rather clinicians who can "think family" and utilize
a variety of family interventions. In my experience also, this is
a more realistic and achievable goal for family therapy training
in most programs.

    4. The authors' model allows for the use of developmental
concepts in relation to the theories of learning which underlie
the three family treatment approaches. This is very important for
child psychiatry residents who, in my experience, benefit a great
deal from appreciating the interrelationship between developmental
concepts and family therapy. I wish that Dr. Grunebaum and
Dr. Chasin had extended the developmental aspects of learning
even further and perhaps they do in their seminar. For example,
Piaget's developmental view of cognition sheds light on the power
of nonverbal communication in therapy, individual or family, and
on the nature of the double bind.

    5. Finally, as the authors emphasize, consideration of the
experiential-existential perspective and the lack of differentiation
seen in family members, facilitates the process of teaching residents about the links between family systems and individual psychodynamics. Helping residents to understand the problems which family
members have in differentiating of necessity involves teaching
about the separation-individuation developmental process, attachment, separation and loss psychology, and the mechanism of projective identification. These links between individual, dynamic,
intrapsychic issues and the phenomena observed in family systems is
critical, in my experience, to being able to effectively integrate
family therapy training into dynamic child psychaitry training.

    This leads me to one of the possible problems with Dr. Grune-
baum and Dr. Chasin's conceptual framework. Like any conceptual
framework that attempts to cover a broad range of clinical issues
and to span diverse, conceptual and theoretical perspectives, it

must of necessity schematize complex issues and, therefore, runs
the risk of over-simplification. I believe that this is the case in
relation to several aspects of the three treatment approaches
described. For example, I was surprised that in relation to
learning through imitation and identification and the treatment
appoach of modeling, the authors do not mention corrective emotional
and object relationship experience which has long been recognized
as significant in psychotherapeutic change in both adults and
children. As I have stressed elsewhere (Malone, 1979), corrective
emotional experience is particularly important in family therapy
and provides another important link between family therapy and
dynamic psychotherapy. Object relations theory addresses this issue
in its concern with the way in which children internalize their
parents as models and how these models influence and are influenced
by subsequent relations with significant others in the environment.
In attempting to correct maladaptive inner models, psychoanalytic
methods of therapy rely on the relearning that occurs through the
transference--the patient's distortions of the therapist are
connected with the earlier parental and sibling relationships
with whom the models were first developed. In family therapy the
affects, attitudes, and behavior of the therapist which are
observed and experienced by family members as he reacts and interacts with them are very powerful and often more important and
effective than what he says. Instead of being inducted, provoked,
or stimulated to react or interact as expected, following and
repeating the pathological patterns of the family, the therapist
provides a different relationship experience which can serve to
correct maladaptive inner models. Importantly, in the treatment
of children, family therapy offers a means of producing actual
change in the parents through their own corrective experience and
identification with the model of the therapist. Thus, the model
of parent-child interaction changes, directly producing a much
more powerful corrective experience for the child.

Along similar lines, in the authors' discussion of treatment,
the separation of insight, changed behavior, and new and mutative
emotional experience seems schematic and more than a bit artificial
to me. In my experience, each of these aspects of therapeutic
change usually interact with each other in a reciprocal fashion.
Insight must involve some change in behavior--e.g., symptomatic
behavior or acting out behavior--and often leads to new and
mutative emotional experience. Similarly, changed behavior often
stems from or leads to new and mutative emotional experience and
vice versa and either may lead to insight.

One possible problem which the conceptual framework can lead
to, which is a welcome one, is the demand it places on residents.
Teaching residents that different theoretical perspectives are
equally and simultaneously valid is appealing, but it is also
demanding. Dr. Grunebaum and Dr. Chasin expect residents to master

several theoretical perspectives, to carry out careful diagnostic assessments, and to have skill in using a range of techniques to accomplish therapeutic goals. This is asking a lot of residents. However, in my experience, any thoughtful and serious effort to integrate family therapy training into a dynamically oriented residency must demand a lot of the residents <u>and</u> the faculty. Dr. Grunebaum and Dr. Chasin are to be congratulated for aiming so high in a training program which they do not control.

REFERENCES

Malone, C. A. Child psychiatry and family therapy: An Overview. <u>Journal of the American Adademy of Child Psychiatry</u>, 1979, <u>18</u>: 4-21.

HOW DOES THE FAMILY'S LEVEL OF DEVELOPMENT INFLUENCE THE THERAPIST'S

APPROACH?   GENERAL DISCUSSION

DR. CHRIST

The family's level of development would appear to influence the therapist's approach. With families who have younger children, you might have to use a different approach than if you have a family with older adolescents. If you have families who are, for example, concrete operational in their thinking capacity, but are not formal operational, would you use one approach versus another? In other words, would the level of cognitive development of the family influence your choice of theoretical perspectives or treatment approaches?

DR. GRUNEBAUM

I think that is a very important question. I do not know that I have the answer to it at this point. In my paper, I spoke about Loevinger's view that an intervention in the family can be viewed through multiple perspectives and experienced by the family in multiple different ways. When treatment is not progressing, it is very often precisely because the therapist is being experienced in a certain way, or the therapist interventions are being experienced in a way which are not being thought about at that particular point.

Further, I do believe that there are stages in the treatment of families. Thus, for instance, we allude to one, namely that it is important in most instances for the family therapist to make some effort to try to have the members of the family feel understood early in therapy, and most family therapists want to try to understand what it feels like for each person to be in the room. I think that is almost a prerequisite for beginning work with a family. Jay Haley contends that this can be accomplished in the first five or ten minutes of an interview, but I must say it takes me a good deal longer.

Charismatic therapists like Elvin Semrad and Sal Minuchin have the ability to establish this bond very quickly. It was

impressive for those of you who had heard Elvin Semrad do this in
the initial five or ten minutes of the interview, and soon the
patient was talking about things that no one dreamt a patient
could have talked about in less than several years of intensive
therapy. But I think most of us have to operate in the ways
that suit our personalities, which means often that we are slower,
more pedestrian, and that we approach things more gradually. We
need to be good workmen--craftsmen, not magicians, and I think
there is a staging operation to the kinds of interpretations and
insights that one offers, naturally depending a great deal on
the child's level of cognitive development.

One of the discomforts of many family therapists who are
not trained as child psychiatrists is that they are simply
scared to death of anyone who does not talk, and talk logically
to boot, and so they will not work with children. They do not
have the sense of what you can learn with a child, even a newborn
baby in a mother's arms. What you can learn is what is going on
in that family by how that baby is handled. But I do think
therapists are moving in that direction. Clearly, we are going
to end up with a critical problem and challenge. If family
therapy is as important as I believe it is, and most of you
believe it is, then one cannot train adult psychiatrists who are
unable to work with children. This importance takes on greater
significance in the light of Allan Gurman and Kniskern's monograph
on research in family therapy. They conclude that we are now
past the stage where the family therapist has to demonstrate the
effectiveness of family and couples therapy. In fact, it is
incumbent upon the individual therapist to demonstrate that
individual therapy does not have destructive effects on other
members of the family than the member who is being treated.

DR. FLOMENHAFT

You tried to differentiate among the different family therapy
models, i.e. Bowen, Boszormeny-Nagy, etc. What are some of the
implications for training out of these different approaches to
family therapy?

DR. GRUNEBAUM

It seems to me one of the problems with family therapy is
that Bowen has his theory, Nagy has his theory, and Minuchin and
Satir have their theory and so forth and so on. And one of our
efforts is to try to tease out from these theories those elements
which can be classified under broader categories than simply the
name of the person whose theory it is. Our effort is to try to
look at these theories in such a way that one can see what it is
that Nagy and Bowen hold in common. Thus, Bowen, for instance,

sends people home to talk to their family members to differentiate themselves from their families of origin. This is similar to a Nagian journey into earlier loyalties. Bowen might well repudiate that idea.

To take another case in point: If you re-read, as I did recently, Minuchin's publications it is very clear that while Minuchin, in his own words, is a structuralist, in his book and on tape he is eminently experiential and unusually adept at getting into the family and getting them to accept him. And there is a moral dimension to his writings which does not always come across in his tapes. So we have engaged in an effort to tease out of what else is Minuchin saying in this structural intervention. What are the identification aspects of a highly authoritarian structural intervention? Or what are the structural and experiential aspects of an interpretation and of the interpretation approach? To think about it in this broader way permits one to get away from names and into the commonalities and differences of approaches, interventions, and techniques.

AUDIENCE MEMBER

There is often a temptation among residents in child psychiatry to allow the age of the children in the family to become determining factors as to which intervention is used. If they have very young children who are not capable of carrying out a lot of secondary thought processing or are involved in a lot of play, then the residents make a short-cut. The resident feels that the historical perspective is not appropriate because these children will only be able to process a behavioral perspective. I would like to hear you comment on how one deals with that particular problem which is really common with child psychiatry trainees?

DR. GRUNEBAUM

First of all, the entire family certainly needs to be present for an evaluation. What one then does, and how one wishes to work with people will depend on many different factors. There is very often a temptation with a young child to work with the parents and not work with the child. That may be useful, but at some point, it may again be useful to work with the child and the parents together. How the individual stages and thinks about the therapy are the critical elements and not only who is present in the room. I do think you are correct that there is a certain reluctance on the part of trainees in child psychiatry as well as trainees in adult psychiatry to have young people around who do not talk, and who run around and create havoc. In part, it also depends upon one having some understanding of young children and how one's office is equipped and set up. I do not think there is a simple answer to this sort of thing.

FAMILY THERAPY AND CHILD PSYCHIATRY TRAINING: ISSUES, PROBLEMS AND
STRATEGIES

Charles A. Malone, M.D.

Case Western Reserve University

Cleveland, Ohio

INTRODUCTION

It is very timely to have this symposium on Family Therapy
in the Training of Child Psychiatrists. Effective integration of
family therapy into child psychiatry training is an extremely
challenging task with which many child psychiatric educators have
struggled for a number of years. The task has been complicated and
made more difficult by the unfortunate conflict and polarization
between child psychiatry and family therapy (Brown, 1972;
McDermott and Char, 1974; Malone, 1974). In the past, and even
currently, dynamically oriented child psychiatrists have opposed
or resisted family therapy on the grounds that it interferes with
transference and needed confidentiality in child therapy, and that
it subjected children to the potentially traumatic effects of being
overtly confronted with the covert dangers in their intrafamilial
lives. Family therapists, on the other hand, have opposed or
rejected dynamic child psychiatry on the grounds that isolated
treatment of children ignores the sources of their disturbance
in pathological family patterns, in marital discord, and in the
parent's own problems.

While the polarization between dynamic child psychiatry and
family therapy still persists and must be confronted in any serious
effort to integrate family therapy into child psychiatry training,
fortunately, it no longer dominates the relationship between the
two fields as it once did. On the contrary, many, if not most,
child psychiatrists and family therapists have been able to move
beyond dichotomous polemics and to take a middle position in which
intrapsychic dynamics and interpersonal transactions and the interventions related to them are seen as interrelated and interdepend-

ent. The central concept involved is the inseparability of internal
and external—that a child or adolescent cannot be accurately understood or treated apart or in isolation from his meaningful life
contexts: family, school, peers and neighborhood (Malone, 1974).
According to this view (Malone, 1979) while conflicts which may
provide the basis for later pathology arise in the first place in
interactions with the demands and prohibitions of the parents,
it would be an error to ignore the fact that children interact
with parents on the strength of their individual characteristics
and innate endowment (Freud, 1972). Similarly, children should
not be assessed or treated without taking family influences into
account; without knowledge of the impact of family influences,
neither the child's developmental successes or failures, nor his
adjustments or maladjustment will be seen in their true light
(Freud, 1972). Psychological development and functioning are seen
as a reciprocal intergenerational family process. Families even
develop patterns in which members share the same personality
characteristics, coping styles, prejudices, defense mechanisms and
symptom clusters when they fall psychiatrically ill (Anthony, 1973).

Despite the polarization which has existed, increasingly child
psychiatrists and other child mental health professionals have
used family therapy in their clinical practice and discovered its
valuable application to a wide range of clinical tasks. As a
result of this increased use of family therapy in child mental
health services the need for and the demand for family therapy
training in child psychiatry training programs has been on the rise
in recent years. Realizing that combining the complementary
features of family therapy and dynamic child psychiatry offers
invaluable advantages and opportunities in the clinical practice
of child psychiatry, child psychiatry programs have in increasing
numbers undertaken the arduous task of integrating family therapy
into their core curriculum. Increasingly, programs have recognized
that family therapy not only has a role in child psychiatry
training, but that it is or should be a central and essential
element.

PLACE OF FAMILY THERAPY IN CHILD PSYCHIATRY TRAINING

As welcome and desirable as this change is, child psychiatry
training programs committed to integrating family therapy into
their core curriculum are confronted with a number of significant
educational problems. This leads me to the purpose of this paper.
Given the fact that without an integrated family therapy component,
child psychiatry training would be incomplete and skewed, what
are the general issues and problems that are likely to be encountered and what teaching methods can be employed to address
them effectively?

The heart of the training matter centers around the task of combining and integrating the complementary features of dynamic child psychiatry and family therapy. In order to accomplish this goal, a child psychiatry training program must recognize and systematically address the following four areas: the real and imagined sources of polarization between child psychiatry and family therapy, the diverse often competing "schools" of family therapy and the proliferation of techniques which has resulted from preoccupation with experimentation in therapeutic technique (Ackerman, 1972), the lack of a unifying theory of family therapy and of a systematic body of knowledge regarding family diagnosis and dynamics which can be related to what is known regarding individual psychology, and, most importantly, the need to enable residents to become "bilingual," that is, to be able to understand, use clinically, and speak the "language" of child development and intrapsychic dynamics <u>and</u> the "language" of transactional process, family dynamics and the family as a psychosocial system.

Reaching these objectives poses a sizeable, if not monumental, challenge for child psychiatry educators. It involves developing a sequence of seminars, clinical conferences and supervised clinical work that will provide a sound knowledge base in relation to both family and individual psychology and that will develop interviewing skills in relation to individual children and parents, the parents as a parental or marital couple, family subsystems, and the family as a whole that can be employed in diagnostic, treatment and consultative services.

The development of such a curriculum requires the training program to have a broad flexible base in its conceptual and theoretical orientation and to operate in relation to a range of inpatient, outpatient and consultation services which, at least to a substantial degree, combine work with individuals, couples, family subsystems and the family as a whole. Above all, it requires a faculty which can accept and be committed to integrating the complemental features of dynamic child psychiatry and family therapy despite the range of individual talents and interests required for broad based child psychiatry training. These requirements, which place a considerable demand on the faculty and the service facility, are not easily met. Even when these requirements are met, however, the success of the program remains problematic because the expectation that residents will become "bilingual" is so extremely difficult to achieve. Since a significant number of child psychiatry residents do not become that fluent in their "native" dynamic, developmental, intrapsychic "language," the expectation that residents will become bilingual must be placed in a realistic perspective. The expectation that residents will develop skill in both individual and family diagnosis, treatment, and consultation must be viewed as a very difficult goal to achieve--one that involves a number of problems for faculty and

student alike. Before turning to curriculum content and design,
let me describe some of the common problems which appear in this
more complex and demanding training endeavor.

COMMON PROBLEM AREAS

     While integrating family therapy into the core child psychiatry
curriculum offers many important and far-reaching advantages, it
also presents problems and disadvantages. To begin with, since
family therapy lacks a unified theory, it is difficult to integrate
the various diverse, fragmentary, often competing theories of
family treatment with each other and even more difficult to
integrate them with the dynamic and developmental concepts of
child psychiatry. Thus, this type of training lacks a clear-cut
well established theoretical model that explicates the interrelationship between transactional process and individual psychology.
As a consequence, residents do not have a well organized conceptual
framework to provide guidelines in their clinical work and to
assist them in becoming bilingual.

     The clinical tasks involved in combining the complementary
features of dynamic child psychiatry and family therapy confront
residents and faculty with the arduous task of applying a wide
range of techniques, without benefit of a unified theory,
depending on clinical indications. This presents a significant
challenge to professional competence for the residents and their
supervisors. The challenge to professional competence and the
complexity of the conceptual issues coupled with the pain and
frustration of the clinical task of diagnosing and treating serious
child, adolescent, adult, marital and family psychopathology often
leads to defensive disengagement and polarization. Moving to a
polar position in the individual analytic versus family systems
controversy is a tempting alternative for residents or supervisors which can be used as a defense or protection against the
personal or interpersonal stress they are under. Polarization to
one theoretical/conceptual model is usually coupled with intellectualization and rationalization as the merits of one approach versus
another are argued, while the underlying sources of stress are
avoided and ignored. A particularly important issue for residents
in the resolution of the stress experienced in training involves
the degree to which they may attempt to escape from the rigors,
vicissitudes, and growing pains of understanding and working with
intrapsychic conflict and pain. While family therapy techniques
make direct exploration of intrapsychic derivatives at the level
of interpersonal process possible, they also make avoidance of
intrapsychic conflict possible through efforts to achieve results
solely through environmental manipulation. The compliance of many
families in this bypassing of the more painful course of struggling
with intrapsychic pain is predictable and leads to "results" which

may be mis-interpreted as successful treatment (Malone, 1974).

The integration of family therapy into a child psychiatry training program must be consistently and effectively supported by various organizational and educational structures. In terms of teaching, supervision plays a key role. Consequently, problems around supervision are apt to occur and must be given prompt and continuing attention. Confronted by the difficult clinical and conceptual tasks involved in this type of training, child psychiatry residents depend more heavily than usual on their supervisors. Lacking a well established theoretical model, residents may experience professional identity and professional role strain and hence rely more on their supervisors as role models. The issue of professional identity and role may be compounded, if the supervision and teaching of family therapy is entirely or predominantly carried out by psychologists or social workers and not by child psychiatrists who are family therapists. In addition, if family therapy supervision by psychologists or social workers is complicated by interdisciplinary competition and territoriality, the problems may become extreme and disruptive to the program. Similarly, if the supervisors of family therapy have been trained in different "schools" of family treatment and "push" their brand of family therapy exclusively, the net result is likely to be confusing and disruptive rather than enriching. In terms of experiencing family therapy as an integral part of child psychiatry, residents usually need to observe and be supervised by child psychiatrists who do family therapy as well as individual child and adolescent psychotherapy. In addition, where family therapy is combined with individual child or parent therapy or couple treatment, problems may arise if supervision does not rest in the hands of the child psychiatrist/family therapy supervisor. Splitting of the clinical work along individual versus family lines is apt to occur where there are two supervisors, one for the individual treatment and the other for the family treatment, particularly if each supervisor is not skilled in doing and supervsing both family and individual treatment. Since the combining of treatments poses difficult clinical, technical, and conceptual issues, supervision by one person optimizes the residents' exposure to the clinical thinking and judgment that must go into the process of interrelating the content of the concomitant individual, couple and family treatment. Such supervisory experiences, in fact, offer the optimal ground for the residents' learning to become "bilingual."

Closely related to the broad range of clinical tasks involved when family therapy is combined with individual or couple treatment, is the problem of changing focus and technique depending on the dynamics of the family subsystem being seen. In family therapy transference and counter-transference issues may be dealt with quite differently than they are in individual treatment.

In family therapy, the focus is on stimulating and promoting transactional processes around unresolved conflicts rather than on one-to-one exchanges with the therapist which are so central to individual therapy. The amount of activity--physical, emotional, and interpersonal--required of the therapist in family therapy is much greater than in individual therapy. Combining individual treatment with family therapy imposes on residents the necessity of utilizing transference and countertransference, the focus of the interventions, and their own activity differently in individual as compared to family therapy. This task of "shifting gears" is a difficult one to master and places extra demands on the residents and their supervisors.

Ironically, the very power of family therapy also presents a problem for residents. The rapidity with which data are collected and conflict is uncovered may be threatening to trainees who are unready or unable to join the family in working toward conflict resolution. This places increased emphasis on the well known and ubiquitous training task of helping trainees to acknowledge and work through (in their own treatment, if needed) their personal blocks to recognizing and responding to the needs of their patients (Malone, 1974).

The need for self awareness is particularly necessary in relation to transference and countertransference issues. While the context and techniques of family therapy may tend to discourage transference phenomena, they appear quite readily and are utilized differently than they are in individual psychotherapy. Transference is of vital significance in the actualization of past conflict and in the correction of inner models of self and others in insight oriented individual treatment. In family therapy, however, transference is mainly used to underscore the manner in which use of or reaction to a therapist repeats or reflects family patterns. Countertransference, on the other hand, occurs much more readily in family therapy than it does in individual therapy. This requires residents to be keenly aware of their own feelings and reactions as they experience themselves being drawn into family patterns. Unless residents are aware of the pull of the expectations of family members, they will not be able to provide a corrective experience or to use countertransference phenomena to demonstrate to the family the nature and power of its complementary patterns.

CURRICULUM CONTENT AND DESIGN

Having provided a general framework, let me now discuss more specifically some of the ways child psychiatry training programs can systematically address the issues and problems regarding family

therapy training which I have outlined. To begin with, I would
stress the importance of the training program having a clear
philosophy and a realistic set of goals. From the outset and
throughout training, the integrated viewpoint described earlier
must be clearly articulated and translated in the organization
and content of the program; the polarization between dynamic
child psychiatry and family therapy must be recognized and
countered. The residents from the time of their recruitment must
be committed to an integrated view and must be helped to appreciate
the sources of the polarization and the expectable difficulties they
will encounter in an integrated program. The residents must be
encouraged to appreciate that the various theories of family
therapy are difficult to integrate with each other and with the
dynamic metapsychological and developmental concepts of child
psychiatry. They must appreciate that being able to recognize and
understand the reciprocal influence of the intrapsychic developmental needs of individual members and the transactional patterns
of the family system is an extremely difficult task.

In view of the complex and difficult nature of the task, it
is important for the faculty and residents to engage in a mutually
supportive realistic endeavor. In this regard, it is useful in the
early phases to deemphasize learning to be a family therapist
and to encourage the residents to learn family subsystem and whole
family interviewing skills and to develop a family orientation
which is reflected in their sensitivity and perceptiveness regarding
transactional process and family patterns, dynamics and developmental issues. At the same time, in supervision, conferences, and
seminars, the residents are regularly exposed to video tapes from
their own and the faculty's clinical work which illustrate the
use of family interviewing in relation to intake, diagnosis,
treatment, and consultation, and which provide shared clinical
experience around which the reciprocal influence of the family
system and the dynamic and developmental needs of individual family
members can be taught. In this process, only the seminar can be
systematic and provide selected video tapes to correlate with
assigned readings in order to promote group discussion of particular
issues. In supervision and conferences, however, the clinical
material is unselected and faculty and residents must explore
issues in a less organized more spontaneous manner. While less
systematic, learning in relation to unselected clinical experiences
has many advantages: it reflects more accurately the realities of
clinical work; it provides a ground for faculty and residents to
explore issues and to experience clinical discoveries together;
and, finally, the spontaneous engagement of faculty with clinical
issues allows residents to share in their thinking and to gain a
more realistic appraisal of and respect for clinical accumen.
In this regard, I might point out that I am generally opposed to
the use of edited training tapes designed to demonstrate clinical
skills and therapeutic techniques because they often present an

unrealistic, virtuoso performance view of clinical work and offer
models which appear beyond the residents' reach and which are more
often imitated than learned.

As important and valuable as spontaneous exploration and
discovery are in the learning process, the training program must
be clearly and well structured, including structures which
encourage spontaneity, exploration, discovery and the activity
of the residents in the learning process. To begin with, there
must be a clear institutional commitment to and support for the
integrated program at the level of the Division of Child Psychiatry
and the Departmentof Psychiatry which is reflected in and supported
by the child and adolescent psychiatry service delivery system.
Since the faculty will not be equally bilingual, it is essential
to have a cadre of child psychiatrist-family therapists on the full-
time faculty to serve as key teachers and core supervisors for
the residents. This ensures that the residents will work most
closely and intensively with faculty who are models of an integrated
approach, who can teach play therapy, individual psychotherapy,
marital and family therapy separately and in combination and who,
as core supervisors, can assist the residents in the task of
integrating the components of family psychology with the components
of individual dynamic developmental psychology which they are
learning. The family therapy supervision and teaching by this
cadre of child psychiatrists can be augmented and enriched, but
not replaced or superceded by well qualified psychologists, social
workers, or nurses. In supervision, the core supervisors can use
literature and the residents' ongoing clinical work to teach
component skills, to practice translation from dynamic, developmental, intrapsychic language into the language of family dynamics
and transactional process and vice versa. The presence of
bilingual child psychiatrist-family therapy supervisors can
facilitate the effectiveness of other teachers in the training
program. Thus, faculty members with expertise in specific areas
such as cognitive development, psychopharmacology, pediatric
neurology, group therapy, school consultation or behavior
modification can be utilized optimally even though they are not
family therapists and the area in which they teach is not or may
not be directly related to family therapy.

As critical as the supervisory process is to the whole
training outcome, it must be supported and reenforced by clinical
assignments, conferences, and seminars. The didactic-clinical
seminar on family therapy is most important. Utilizing assigned
readings and illustrative video tapes, the family therapy seminar
can systematically address the task of teaching fundamental
concepts, reviewing the writing of leading exponents of family
therapy, and presenting in an objective manner the various "schools"
of family therapy. In doing this, the seminar leader must

explicitly avoid polemics and encourage and open exploration of
the field in which sound and useful ideas, principles, and concepts,
and techniques are identified and related to clinical issues.
Without erasing the important differences that exist in the thinking
and practices among leading exponents of family therapy, the
seminar leader draws attention to the common conceptual and technical elements that are present. An effort is made to increase
the residents' understanding the multiple clinical approaches which
characterize the field may not, in fact, represent distinct forms
of treatment. Residents are taught to categorize techniques
according to therapeutic goals and that the same technique--e.g.
the use of tasks--can be used as a paradoxical directive or as a
means of increasing awareness and insight, depending on how it is
used.

     Using unedited videotaped applications of family interviewing
to a range of clinical tasks, the seminar group identifies salient
family process phenomena and important family therapy concepts.
Videotapes are also used to develop observational and tracking
skills so that residents become able to identify family patterns
and diagnose family problems in terms of relationship and role,
structure, communication, dynamic, and developmental issues.
Based on observations and discussion of videotapes, the residents
are asked to formulate a family diagnosis and to diagram the
relationship and role structure of the family. The seminar group
is then asked to translate the family diagnosis into individual
dynamic and developmental terms and to identify treatment goals
based on the combined individual and family diagnostic formulations.
Throughout the illustrative videotape components of the seminar,
the leader repeatedly attempts to combine the clinical phenomena
which illustrate individual dynamic developmental concepts with
the transactional process phenomena which illustrate family
system dynamics.

     Since the central objective of the training program is to
develop child psychiatric clinicians who are able to understand
and integrate the complemental features of family therapy and
dynamic child psychiatry, it is critical that the program offers
multiple opportunities for the residents to recognize, experience
and learn the complementary links between the two fields. Therefore, from the outset and throughout their training, the residents
must be exposed to and learn about the contributions which the
two fields can make to each other. In their ongoing clinical
work, they must experience how family therapy broadens their
diagnostic and therapeutic range; how it provides a deeper understanding of psychological development and functioning, of conflict
and symptom formation, of the intergenerational transmission of
impulses, attitudes, conflicts and defenses, and of the process
of therapeutic change. Equally important, residents must experience
how dynamic child psychiatry broadens the scope and effectiveness

of family therapy through understanding and appropriately utilizing
the play, fantasy and verbalization of children and by building
bridges between dynamic developmental concepts and family therapy
--bridges which can provide unifying themes, thereby reducing some
of the confusion and fragmentation created by diverse techniques.
In this latter process, residents gain an appreciation for the
value of dynamic developmental insights in making sense out of the
complex data involved in family transactions, in judging the indications or contraindications for family therapy, in choosing
between alternative intervention strategies, and in achieving some
degree of order in their thinking about the multiple diverse
approaches used in family treatment.

CONTRIBUTIONS OF FAMILY THERAPY TO CHILD PSYCHIATRY

        Clinical conferences and the residents' ongoing supervised
clinical experience should provide a solid basis for learning the
usefulness of family therapy in diagnosis and treatment and its
applicability to a variety of clinical tasks. In relation to
diagnosis, the residents learn that family interviews enable them
to assess how a child's symptoms or dysfunction are influenced by
and influence the family system. They learn that when family
interaction is skillfully facilitated, the presenting problem
actually happens in the here and now of the family interview.
This offers them an opportunity to observe not only family reactions
and contributions to the problem, but also the balance of capacity
and motivation for or against change in the family as a whole
(Skynner, 1969). This enables them to insure the involvement of
the psychologically relevant family members who collusively or
openly are part of and contribute to the problem, or to avoid at
the outset interminable treatment by working with only part of the
family involved in the problem. Through their own clinical
experience, residents learn that family interviewing is particularly
useful in determining the nonverbal communications which contribute
to a child's problems, in reducing guilt and fear in parents and
children, in bolstering self-esteem, especially in the identified
patient, and in countering loyalty conflicts or secret keeping
that block open communication. They develop increasing skill in
using family interviews to identify characteristic patterns of
communication, affect exchange, and conflict. They gradually
appreciate how family interviewing is particularly useful in
identifying structural imbalance (scapegoating, splitting,
alliances, collusions, symbiotic or sadomasochistic dyads, role
reversal and so on), patterns of projective identification and
underlying marital, parental and family of origin problems (Malone,
1979).

        In relation to treatment, the residents' ongoing supervised
family therapy assists them in learning the many therapeutic

advantages of family approaches in treatment (Malone, 1974).
They come to appreciate that family therapy offers more direct
therapeutic access to acting out and symptomatic behavior. Family
therapy increases the residents' ability to recognize and counter
the secondary gain which the child's symptoms provide for parents,
siblings and the child himself. It increases therapeutic potential
by offering a means of identifying and enlisting healthy members
or aspects of the family. Residents also develop an understanding
of the indications for family therapy as they discover that it is
particularly useful in treating developmental delays and certain
types of presenting problems in children, in modifying relationship
and role imbalance, in dealing with unmourned losses or an actual
or impending family crisis, in countering scapegoating and the
use of the child's symptoms as a conflict detouring mechanism, in
disspelling myths, divisive secret keeping and other chronic intrafamilial communication problems and in working with families
dominated by projective identification or where marital, parental
and/or family of origin problems underlie the child's presenting
problems (Malone, 1974). Most important, in the interest of an
integrated view residents develop an appreciation for the fact
that family therapy is also valuable when combined with individual
therapy in furthering the psychotherapeutic process in relation to
children suffering with moderate to severe intrapsychic problems.
Thus, they come to learn that it can be an invaluable aid in
the treatment of precisely those problems for which analytically
oriented psychotherapy is usually best suited and most effective.

      In training child psychiatrists, however, it is essential to
deal quite openly and directly with the contraindications as well
as the indications for family therapy (Malone, 1979). Residents
must gradually learn that family therapy is not helpful when the
very process of focusing on family transactions intensifies and
perpetuates the pathological patterns within the family without
prospects for repair. This is the case in families where one of
the parents has severe problems and is particularly resistant, and
the rest of the family cannot become involved in treatment without
risking a breakup of the family, which they are unwilling to do.
This is also the case where there is a dominance of sadistic
gratification and destructive behavior in a family such as physical
and psychological abuse and there is not enough discomfort to
motivate the family to change. Similarly while family interviews
and treatment can be very useful in relation to marital separation,
family therapy is not indicated and may be harmful when the
separated or separating parents have an extremely hostile relationship which is set off by each other's presence. When a firm
decision to divorce has been reached, bringing the estranged couple
together in family treatment runs counter to their psychological
task of separating and relinquishing and working through their
ambivalent attachment. Despite this, however, some structured
family interviews may be helpful or necessary when the children

are being caught in the middle of the divorcing couples' continuation of their marital battle (Malone and Gispert, 1977).
While family therapy is often indicated for adolescents with
separation problems, there are times when seeing adolescents with
their parents perpetuates rather than counters pathological
dependency or symbiotic ties (Williams, 1968). Similarly, with
older adolescents preoccupied and in the process of disengaging
and emancipating from the family, family treatment often runs
counter to the adolescent's developmental needs.

COMPLEMENTARY LINKS BETWEEN DYNAMIC CHILD PSYCHIATRY AND FAMILY
THERAPY[1]

In my experience, a critical component of successful
integration of family therapy into child psychiatry training involves the residents learning the various ways in which their
child psychiatry knowledge base and clinical skills are crucial
to the conduct of family therapy. It is extremely important for
them to realize that their emphasis on careful diagnosis, their
appreciation of the child's contribution to his own and the
family's problems, and their knowledge of child development play
a critical role in being able to carry out effective family therapy.
This awareness is primarily developed through training experiences
directed at three areas of learning:

(1) the role of children in family therapy
(2) the application of dynamic developmental concepts
     to core clinical issues in family therapy
(3) the application of dynamic developmental concepts
     to the issue of therapeutic change in family therapy

The Role of Children in Family Therapy

In relation to the role of children in family therapy, child
psychiatry residents must learn from experience how their ability
to talk with young children, school age children and adolescents
and their capacity to understand and utilize the play, fantasy
and verbalizations of children for diagnostic and therapeutic
purposes are very important in the conduct of family therapy. It
is important for residents to appreciate the ramifications of

---

[1]The material presented in this section represents a translation
into training experiences for residents of concepts regarding the
contribution of dynamic child psychiatry to family therapy which
I have written about elsewhere (Malone, 1979).

including children in family therapy. They learn, for example,
that it is essential to include the so-called "well" siblings.
They are needed to point up family problems outside the index
patient and thus to counter the devaluation involved for the child
labelled as the patient in the family. The residents learn that
these children may well have problems in their own right and may,
in fact, be more disturbed than the index patient. On the other
hand, the "well" siblings may be part of a family pattern of
scapegoating or be in a parental child role. On the other hand,
since the index patient and the parents are usually locked
into chronic, repetitive patterns the "well" siblings are often
more independent and objective and, therefore, able to observe and
identify family patterns and problems.

     The residents also learn the advantages of including children
of various ages in family therapy. When children of various ages
are included, residents are able to observe the response of family
members to children at different stages of development. This
contributes valuable information about the difficulties or
resourcefulness of parents and children regarding phasic developmental issues. At the same time, this offers the residents
opportunities to present models of interaction, communication and
response to children with different developmental needs which can
provide possibilities for corrective emotional experiences. The
inclusion of young children naturally leads to focusing on play
and fantasy and their expressive and defensive use (Zilbach et al.,
1972; Skynner, 1976). Residents learn that older children bring
their expertise in the world outside the family and may be able
to "coach" younger siblings in meeting the challenges of school,
neighborhood or peer group.

Dynamic Developmental Concepts in Relation to Core Clinical Issues
in Family Therapy

     Applications of dynamic developmental concepts to core
clinical issues in family therapy occur throughout the resident's
training particularly in supervision. In my experience, however,
this central area of learning needs to be reenforced through a
continuous case seminar. In the continuous case seminar, the
residents and the seminar leader follow the unfolding of a family
treatment using unedited videotapes. The videotaped clinical
material chosen should represent a typical moderately difficult
family treatment carried out by a child psychiatrist with
sufficient competence that the process moves along smoothly, but
does not have virtuoso, tour de force qualities that place the
interventions employed beyond the residents' reach. It is
preferable for the leader not to have any prior knowledge of the
treatment, thus assuring his or her spontaneous involvement in

the clinical process. The detailed sharing of clinical experience
provided by the videotapes offers many meaningful opportunities
to illustrate and reenforce concepts, theory and salient features
of the various "schools" of family therapy identified in the
didactic seminar on family therapy. It also provides opportunity
to further develop observational and tracking skills through
exercises focused on identifying the patterns of role and relationship, communication, problem solving, affect exchange, and
identification in the family with a view to formulating and
diagramming a family diagnosis which identifies structural imbalance, areas of unresolved conflict, communication problems and
dynamic developmental issues. In order to reenforce their
bilingual ability, the residents are encouraged to translate the
main components of family diagnosis into individual dynamic developmental terms and vice versa. The group is then asked to
formulate treatment goals in structural, communications, conflict
resolution, affective, and dynamic developmental terms. As a
next step, the residents and the leader develop a set of treatment
strategies. As the treatment process unfolds, the leader and
the residents discuss diagnostic, technique, and intervention
issues in relation to the previously formulated goals and strategy.
Based on new data that emerge, modifications are made in relation
to diagnostic formulations and treatment goals and strategies.
The spontaneous quality of the shared clinical experience is
invaluable for the leader. The leader thus has genuine discovery
experiences and must actively reformulate his thinking. This
provides an opportunity for the residents to share in the leader's
clinical thinking as the treatment unfolds.

     As the family treatment process unfolds, the continuous case
seminar offers a number of excellent opportunities to learn about
the application of dynamic developmental concepts to core clinical
issues. For instance, important aspects of conflict and defense,
object relations theory, attachment, separation and loss psychology,
and the separation-individuation developmental process can readily
be identified in a family treatment process. This process starts
with the family's focus on a symptomatic child, and, working
backward through a network of projections, displacements and
identifications, reaches the parental, marital, personal and family
of origin problems which underlie the child's symptom picture
and the family's initial concerns. In this process, the seminar
group identifies complementary patterns involving projective
identification (Wynne, 1965; Zinner and Shapiro, 1972), in which
an unwanted part of one parent is projected onto and identified
in a spouse or a child who in turn develops attitudes of behaviors
which complement the projection. The seminar group also attempts
to identify the various ways the parents carry over unresolved
conflicts and losses, organizing views of self and others,
identifications, and roles from their family of origin into
their current family life. Wherever possible, connections are made

between these ghosts from the past and the character of the
marriage, the nature of parental functioning, and the parent, child
and family interaction.

As part of the seminar process, wherever appropriate, the
clinical material is connected with the conceptualizations of
leading family therapists. An effort is made to help residents
to consolidate their understanding of different "schools" of
family therapy and to relate these concepts to clinical phenomena.
Residents achieve some degree of independence from any one "school"
by realizing that leading family therapists describe the same or
similar clinical issues albeit in different language. The
residents learn, for example, that regardless of their theoretical
orientation, many well known figures in the field of family therapy
conceptualize their therapeutic approach in terms of assisting
family members to break pathological symbiotic and dependency ties
and to separate and differentiate themselves from current and
past family enmeshment in order to achieve autonomy and effective
independent functioning. Thus, Bowen (1966) emphasizes the process
of differentiation of spouses from each other and a pathologically
dependent symbiotic-like emotional oneness, while Ackerman and
Behrens (1959) speak of separation and differentiation from the
parental matrix. Satir (1964), while presenting herself to
families as an expert in and teacher of communication, is also
committed to helping each family member experience "individuation."
Boszormenyi-Nagy (1965), who has developed perhaps the most
ambitious integration of object relations theory, ego psychology
and transactional process, has as a cornerstone of his approach
the uncovering of distorted part object introjections and projections of parents within the nuclear family. Finally, Paul
(1967) explicitly organizes family treatment as a process
designed to exorcise the ghosts from the family of origin which
dominate the life of the nuclear family. Paul attempts to uncover
the effects of the unrelinquished object, usually an unmourned
loss of a parent or sibling, on current family life and to carry
out a process of mourning and relinquishing.

The focus of the seminar can then shift to consider some of
the relationships these conceptualizations of family therapy and
object relations theory and the separation-individuation developmental process (Mahler et al., 1975). The residents are asked
to review literature on these subjects (covered in other seminars)
and seminar discussion centers on the way in which children
internalize their family life experience, forming models which
guide current and future behavior. The seminar considers some
aspects of the interrelationship between the internalization of
models and the separation-individuation process. The residents'
attention is drawn to the fact that the development of a full
degree of autonomy means that a person not only has internalized
stable differentiated models of self and other which can be

modified or corrected by experience, but that he has also achieved
a degree of independence and conflict-free functioning which enables
him to meet new situations and people without necessarily having
to repeat inner models. On the other hand, when separation-
individuation is incomplete, the individual's inner models of self
and other are not well differentiated. They are not or may not
be modified or corrected by experience and the individual tends
or is compelled to repeat them. As a byproduct of this discussion,
residents begin to appreciate that incomplete separation-individuation is one of the major indications of family treatment and that
modification of distorted, maladaptive inner models through
corrective object relations experience is one of the major means
of therapeutic change in family therapy.

     The seminar focus now shifts back to the videotape material
and the review of the continuous case and the therapeutic issues
involved in attempting to assist family members to resolve
maladaptive object relations related to developmental deficits in
the separation-individuation process. This usually offers
opportunities to bring attachment, separation and loss psychology
into the picture. As the seminar group considers treatment
issues, it becomes possible to emphasize the reactions and
resistance of family members to change. In dealing with marital/
parental issues, for example, as change occurs and one spouse is
able to differentiate and become more independent that person must
be prepared for distressing reactions in other family members
(Bowen, 1966; Brown, 1969). The most profoundly threatening of
these reactions often involves withdrawal with the implicit or
explicit concomitant threat of separation on the part of his or
her spouse. In response to such a reaction, the treated spouse
is likely to get depressed, confused, and develop a whole spectrum
of physical symptoms (Bowen, 1966). In order to maintain the
change achieved and evolve a new balance in the marriage, the
treated spouse must be able to tolerate the depressive affect and
anxiety engendered by the threatened loss of attachment implicit
in the mate's strong resistance to the change and reaction of
withdrawal.

     Brown (1969) places these issues into a broader perspective
which includes children. He notes that patterns of interpersonal
relationship in families often protect inner models from being
altered by real events. Therefore, significant change in family
members and intrafamilial relationships produces or threatens to
produce a partial internal loss (relinquishing of internal self
and other object representations or models) and is resisted and/or
reacted to with separation anxiety and grief. Thus, Brown points
out, change in a wife engenders anxiety in a husband which may
lead to a new surge of over-involvement with the symptomatic child,
who also reacts to the change in his mother as an actual or

threatened loss and may temporarily regress and become more
infantile and demanding, which in turn reinforces and is reinforced
by the father's over-involvement. These events in turn exert a
strong pull on the wife/mother to return to her old patterns.
Reviewing these issues helps residents to understand that as
family therapists they must anticipate and be prepared to help
family members recognize resistance to change and work through
threatened and actual object relationship losses which are inevitably associated with significant change in family members and
intrafamilial relationships, or else the change will not last or
will not be beneficial to the family. Thus, whatever language
the residents frame their understanding in, they learn that as
family therapists who intend to help the symptomatic child by
removing the influence of underlying marital, parental, or family
of origin problems they must appreciate the psychology of attachment, separation and loss, the relationship between inner models
and external intrafamilial relationships (in both parents and
children), and that resistance to change involves not only a
counterreaction to a shift in the family hemostasis, but expectable
psychological reactions to threatened and actual and object and
part object loss.

Dynamic Developmental Concepts in Relation to Therapeutic Change in Family Therapy

Consideration of the therapeutic issues involved in assisting
families to resolve maladaptive object relations related to
developmental deficits in the separation-individuation process
and the residents' supervised work in family treatment provide many
opportunities to explore applications of developmental and dynamic
concepts to the issue of therapeutic change. This is particularly
true in relation to a corrective emotional and object relationship
experience which has long been recognized as being significant
in psychotherapeutic change in both adults and children (Alexander,
1957). Child psychiatrists who are family therapists have
frequently pointed to the significant advantage of family therapy
in relation to corrective emotional experience in work with
children (Williams, 1968). In relation to supervised individual
psychotherapy, residents learn that children often reproduce
aspects or essential qualities of their troubled or pathological
relationship with a parent. They become increasingly aware of
the ways children project their inner models of self and parent
onto the therapist and the interaction with him or her. Residents
learn to provide corrections of the child's view and experience
of himself by not following the projected model and behaving and
relating differently from the parent. They also learn, however,
that such corrective experiences may be negated or undermined by
the child's continuing intrafamilial experience with the parent
and other family members. Through their own clinical work,

residents gain an understanding that family therapy offers not only
a means of countering the undoing of corrective emotional experience,
but, more importantly, of producing actual change in the parents
(often through their own corrective experience and identification
with the model of the therapist). Thus, the model of parent-child
interaction changes directly, producing a much more powerful
corrective emotional experience.

     The residents' growing appreciation of the role of family
therapy in producing corrective emotional and object relationship
experience leads residents to a fuller consideration of the contro-
versial subject of therapeutic change. In this consideration
residents are encouraged to be concerned not only with change,
but with the process by which it takes place as well. They
gradually realize that change may simply reflect symptom substitu-
tion and that sudden, unprepared-for change may lead to an uncon-
trolled sequence of changes which are harmful to the family. They
know that by avoiding being inducted or provoked to react or inter-
react as expected, following and repeating the pathological
patterns of the family, the therapist provides a different relationship experience which can serve to correct maladaptive intrapsychic
and interpersonal models. They understand that in order to
accomplish this the therapist must feel and recognize nonverbal
behavioral and role expectations which family members project onto
him or her without being taken over by these expectations and
acting out a complementary response which would verify rather than
correct the maladaptive expectation (Skynner, 1976). The residents
also learn that in order to accomplish therapeutic change through
a corrective emotional experience, the therapist must also gently
and sympathetically but firmly counter the avoidance mechanisms
through which family members resist and turn away from the treatment
situation as their anxiety mounts, leaving their expectations
untested and uncorrected.

     In the process of assisting child psychiatry residents to
explore the subject of therapeutic change in relation to family
therapy, it is extremely important that the supervisors and
teachers refer to and utilize dynamic and developmental concepts
where appropriate. It can be pointed out, for example, that in
attempting to correct maladaptive inner models, psychoanalytic
methods of therapy, in contrast with transactional process methods
used in family therapy, rely on the relearning that occurs through
the transference--the patient's distortions of the therapist are
connected with earlier parental and sibling relationships with whom
the models were first developed (Skynner, 1976). Developmental
concepts can be referred to, for example, in considering the powerful effects of nonverbal communication in the corrective process
which occurs in family treatment. Attention can be drawn to
Piaget's cognitive developmental concepts. In Piaget's view, pre-
school, and even young school age children think through concrete

experiential modes rather than symbolic representational ones.
These earlier modes of cognition, also called enactive and iconic,
are not only dominant in early childhood but persist after the
stage of formal operations and advanced symbolic representational
thought are achieved. The concrete experiential modes of cognitive
affective organization are not only developmentally earlier, but
also closer to a person's feelings, drives, bodily sensations,
and preconscious and unconscious mental activity. The residents
are taught that part of the power of nonverbal communication (and
the model of the therapist) stems from its enactive and iconic
quality. It is more readily received because it is less subject
to monitoring by conscious control and defenses organized by
symbolic representation (e.g., intellectualization and rationalization). It "speaks" to those levels of mental activity which
are closer to personal-interpersonal conflict and distortion.
It conveys messages to the mind and the body, informs most in
harmony with the modes of learning of the preschool and early
school age periods of development during which the basic and
most influential inner models of self and others are formed.
Since these inner models are formed mainly through what is
experienced and what is observed, correction of maladaptive
models can occur in a more rapid, direct, and holistic manner
through observing and experiencing the new and more adaptive
model of the therapist. Emphasis on dynamic developmental
concepts in relation to therapeutic change is one of the multiple
ways in which the faculty must teach and demonstrate the complementary relationship between family therapy and dynamic child
psychiatry. Such teaching is, as I have stressed repeatedly
in this paper, crucial to the success of efforts to integrate
family therapy into the core curriculum of child psychiatry
training.

REFERENCES

Ackerman, N. W. The growing edge of family therapy. In:
    C. J. Sager and H. S. Kaplan (Eds.) Progress in Group and
    Family Therapy. New York: Brunner/Mazel, 1972, pp. 44-456.
    _____ and Behrens, M. D. The family group and family therapy.
    In: J. H. Masserman and J. L. Moreno (Eds.) Progress in
    Group and Family Therapy, New York:Grune and Stratton, 1959,
    3:63-78.
Alexander, F. Psychoanalysis and Psychotherapy. London:Ruskin
    House, 1957.
Anthony, E. J. A working model for family studies. In: E. J.
    Anthony and C. Koupernik (Eds.) The Child and His Family,
    New York:Wiley, 1973, 2:3-20.
Boszormenyi-Nagy, I. A theory of relationships. In: I.
    Boszormenyi-Nagy and J. Framo (Eds.) Intensive Family Therapy,
    New York:Harper and Row, 1965, pp. 33-86.

Bowen, M. The use of family therapy in clinical practice.
    Comprehensive Psychiatry, 1966, 7:345-374.
Brown, S. L. Diagnosis, clinical management and family inter-
    viewing. In: J. H. Masserman (Ed.) Science and Psychoanalysis,
    New York:Grune and Stratton, 1969, 14:188-198.
_____Family group therapy. In: B. B. Wolman (Ed.) Manual of Child
    Psychopathology. New York:McGraw-Hill, 1972, pp. 969-10009.
Freud, A. The child as a person in his own right. The Psycho-
    analytic Study of the Child, 1972, 27:621-625.
Mahler, M. S., Pine, F., and Bergmann, A. The Psychological Birth
    of the Human Infant. New York: Basic Books, 1975.
Malone, C. A. Observations on the role of family therapy in child
    psychiatry training. Journal of American Academy of Child
    Psychiatry, 1974, 13:437-458.
_____and Gispert, M. Divorce and the single parent family.
    Read at World Congress of Psychiatry, Honolulu, Hawaii, 1977.
_____ Child psychiatry and family therapy:An overview.
    Journal of American Academy of Child Psychiatry, 1979, 18:
    4-21.
McDermott, J. F. and Char, W. F. The undeclared war between child
    psychiatry and family therapy. Journal of American Academy
    of Child Psychiatry, 1974, 13:422-436.
Paul, N. L. The use of empathy in the resolution of grief.
    Perspectives in Biology and Medicine, 1967, 11:153-169.
Satir, V. Conjoint Family Therapy. Palo Alto:Science and Behavior
    Books, 1964.
Skynner, A.C.R. Indications and contraindications for conjoint
    family therapy. International Journal of Social Psychiatry,
    1969, 15:245-250.
_____ Systems of Family and Marital Psychotherapy. New York:
    Brunner/Mazel, 1976.
Williams, F. S. Family therapy. In: J. Marmor (Ed.) Modern
    Psychoanalysis. Basic Books, 1968, pp. 387-406.
Wynne, L. C. Some indications and contraindications for exploratory
    family therapy. In: I. Boszormenyi-Nagy and J. Framo (Eds.)
    Intensive Family Therapy. New York: Harper and Row, 1965,
    pp. 289-322.
Zilbach, J. J., Bergel, E., and Gass, C. The role of the young
    child in family therapy. In: C. J. Sager and H. S. Kaplan
    (Eds.) Progress in Group and Family Therapy. New York:
    Brunner/Mazel, 1972, pp. 385-399.
Zinner, J. and Shapiro, R. Projective identification as a mode
    of perception and behavior in families of adolescents.
    International Journal of Psychoanalysis, 1972, 53:523-529.

THE SIGNIFICANCE OF A BILINGUAL REPERTOIRE OF PSYCHOLOGICAL THINKING:

DISCUSSION OF DR. MALONE'S PAPER

Saul L. Brown, M.D.

Cedars-Sinai Medical Center

Los Angeles, California

Are we saying things to each other that we already know?
Yes and no. To a large degree, those of us presenting papers
in this symposium are in a group who have evolved somewhat similar
frames of reference drawn from mutually valued theoretical views.
It appears that our relatively small group read similar literature
back in the 1950s and 1960s, cathected similar concepts, and
tried similar clinical interventions. Slowly but somehow
inexorably, our individual experiences have converged in a
conference such as this one. Even our frustrations are convergent,
especially those related to teaching what Charles Malone calls a
"bilingual" repertoire of psychological thinking to child psychiatry
trainees. I would add to this difficulty the one of demonstrating
such thinking to our more experienced colleagues.

Teaching psychoanalysis and child analysis have long been
accepted as an arduous and long term process, extending beyond
the basic training in psychiatry, which in itself is a slow
process. Can this be less true of family therapy? I ask this
only to confront the feeling of discouragement that I and others
sometimes have experienced. Accomplishing the complex weave of
teaching, experiential and clinical experience so lucidly outlined
by Charles Malone requires time, talent, money, and very intense
personal motivation. It requires many individuals helping each
other. Also, it requires a receptive environment--namely, an
academic clinical ecology that is responsive to the various
educational steps he has outlined.

Returning to my question, are we all only saying things to
each other that we already know or are we confronting new issues?
I can easily say that Charles Malone's comments do both for me.

Much of what he says I certainly know or have thought and said
or even written about, but all of us are new enough in our
efforts that we need to repeat ideas to each other so we can
build an enduring educational and theoretical structure. For
example, my interest in the vicissitudes of separation anxiety
dates back not only to my own personal history, but also to
what I thought I understood of my analytic patients early in my
training. However, it was Charles Malone's remarkable description
of his treatment of a ghetto child apropos her covert separation
anxiety, published many years ago, that helped me comprehend how
crucial this particular phenomenon is in the life of a family,
and to see it as a core resistance to both developmental and
therapeutic change.

I believe Dr. Malone's emphasis upon use of unedited tapes
done by relatively inexperienced trainees to be a most valuable
notion. In our center we have done such taping but have not
always used them in the systematic way that Dr. Malone urges. As
he noted, the phenomenon of awe when trainees watch a virtuoso,
often coupled with a kind of passivity in the observers, is best
avoided when the interviewer who is being observed is somewhat
inexperienced. I too have recognized a tendency in observers to
react to the subtle sequences of interactions and process in a
family interview that is done by an expert as if they were
inevitable, not realizing how the expertise of the clinician
contributed to that "inevitability." Errors made by an inexperienced interviewer introduce freshness to the observational
process and evoke the tension necessary for learning. I admit
that Charles Malone's emphasis creates a degree of tension in me
since I am aware of a reluctance to give up the comfortable and
often gratifying role of showing off my clinical technique.
However, I am sure he would settle for doing both kinds of teaching.

The important principles that underly the preceding are
really those of observing clinical work; and of observed and
carefully critiqued experiential learning. Both were too long
neglected in the training of psychiatrists and psychotherapists.
The video-taping system has provided us with a break-through in
clinical education, as has the one-way observation mirror.
However, it is my private belief that most of the early initiative
and courage in the field of clinical psychiatry to be observed
and filmed or video-taped was limited to those clinicians who were
the pioneers in family therapy. People like Ackerman, Bowen,
Jackson, Alger, Minuchin, and others were willing to reveal both
their skills and their awkwardnesses to sophisticated clinicians
and to take their chances! Some others of us have followed close
behind and, I should emphasize, have learned enormously from the
experience of being observed and critiqued. Too many clinicians
who are also teachers have failed to experience this. Of course,

it has not felt <u>quite</u> so comfortable when we've been <u>rejected</u> by
those observing us--especially by our colleagues in child psychiatry. I say that because few of us 15 years ago really expected
dyed-in-the-wool adult psychiatrists and psychoanalysts, deeply
imbedded in dyadic technique and theory, to view family therapy
in a benign way. But child psychiatrists had long been tuned
into family dynamics and the intricate process of how intrapsychic dynamisms are acted-out in the parent-child relationship.
Szurek and Johnson among others long ago provided clear and well
thought out case illustrations showing how the internal psychodynamics of parents were in constant oscillation with the
symptomatic behavior of their children. However, most senior
child psychiatrists were reluctant to observe or apply what they
observed in the new modality of family therapy. I take the
liberty to speculate that here as in other kinds of resistance
to innovation, separation anxiety was at work--the anxiety that
occurs when one lets go of cherished viewpoints and of what one
has felt to be tried and true.

I have no improvements to offer to Dr. Malone's outstanding
paper. He and I are both integrators. We are not out to
establish an either-or confrontation with anyone. But as we all
know, integration is humanity's most vexing challenge. In our
own professional microcosm, integration of our understanding about
intrapsychic mechanisms with our comprehension of transactional
processes in families; and the integration of therapeutic skills
applicable to both individual patients and to families requires
a great amount of learning. Becoming "bilingual" as Dr. Malone
defines it requires respect for and comprehension of several
levels of theoretical formulation, most of which Dr. Malone
alluded to. A certain kind of talent is needed for that. Also
sequential learning is crucial.

In alluding to the temptation to polarize into adversary
theorizing, I believe Dr. Malone is referring to the concerns
raised by some child psychiatrists that family therapy in its
preoccupation with systems theory loses track of individual
psychopathology. In an effort to avoid this danger some years
ago, I found value in thinking about how both therapeutic change
<u>and</u> developmental change may be met by field resistance in the
family system. In other words, the way in which a family system
functions so as to resist the inevitable changes occurring in
individual and family life. Beginning with a basic assumption,
that change is indeed inevitable, a therapist needs to comprehend
what factors are responsible for such resistance to change. As
he begins the search, using family interviews as his medium, it
soon becomes evident whether the balance of factors resisting
change are to be found mainly in the way family sub-systems
are organized or whether mainly in the individual intrapsychic
organization of the named patient or of others in the family.

What this frame of reference does is lead us toward addressing
first things first. Sometimes what needs to be addressed first in
a clinical situation is individual psychopathology; sometimes it
is intrafamilial communication; sometimes it is simple ignorance
on the part of the parents; sometimes it is marital discord;
sometimes it is familial structure; sometimes it is economic
stress; and so on. Thus, family therapy as I have come to view
it and as I believe Dr. Malone has, encompasses many possibilities
for clinical intervention. Unquestionably, it must bow to the
supervening clinical reality affecting a patient at a given time.
Resistance to therapeutic change, when it is a function of field
resistance in the family system requires family system interventions. When resistance to change is a function of individual
psychopathology, individual psychotherapy is indicated. Often,
most often in child psychiatry, shifts from one to the other and
back occur. The organizing principle is resistance to change--
resistance in the family field and in the individuals. This
then becomes systems theory linked to individual psychopathology
and intelligent case management.

     I believe what I have just outlined fits into what
Dr. Malone has provoked us to think about and can be demonstrated
and learned by many, but not all, students of child psychiatry,
using the educational approaches he has outlined. A philosophy
of therapy in a teaching environment is an ideal, personified and
embodied in the senior faculty.

THE DEMANDING TASK OF INTEGRATING FAMILY THERAPY INTO A

CURRICULUM: GENERAL DISCUSSION

AUDIENCE MEMBER

As part of training in some family therapy centers, the
supervisor early on in the treatment actually comes in and joins
the therapist in a session. I have experienced that myself and
found it to be very useful. I wonder if you could comment on
that as a technique of supervision.

DR. MALONE

I did not really go into some of the techniques of supervision.
In my experience, the fastest way to learn effectively is a co-
therapy arrangement with a more experienced person. The yield in
terms of learning is particularly high if that person not only
has a good deal of clinical skill, but is also effective at what
he or she does in conceptualizing family therapy. Clinical and
conceptual skill do not always go together. There are some
marvelous clinicians who have difficulty conceptualizing what they
are doing; there are some marvelous conceptualizers who never do
therapy or cannot do therapy. A more effective and intimate way
of teaching develops when the supervisor joins the resident in
co-therapy of a family.

Personally, I am not keen on the "bug in the ear" and the
telephone on the wall to call people out. Now, sometimes, you
really have to call the supervisee out to rescue a situation you
are observing through a one-way mirror, particularly, when the
excessive distress of the family or the therapist is not being
recognized.

If there is no urgency, however, I prefer to talk about it
with the resident afterwards in a supportive way if it has been
a distressing session, and then to review it in detail.

I find video tapes in many ways more useful for supervision,
though you miss something when you are not in the room. If you
work together with the resident well, you can capture a lot from

reviewing video tapes. You have an added advantage if you can
save a series of tapes. In order to evaluate the progress of both
the trainees and the family, it is very nice to have some base lines
of earlier interviews both from the standpoint of the quality
of the interview in terms of the techniques and the understanding
demonstrated by the resident, as well as where the family was
at that point. Obviously, the later tapes can show the movement
the family makes and the movement that the resident is making in
his or her comprehension of what is going on and how the family
is being treated. The clinical and didactic seminars are very
important because both ways of teaching reinforce in a structured
way what the residents are learning. But the bulk of the learning
takes place in the supervisory process.

I want to make something clear in case it did not come through.
I very much believe in having an interdisciplinary training faculty.
When I stress the role of the child psychiatrist family therapists,
however, it is because if they are absent from the program, then
the model that the residents have is that child psychiatrists only
do individual therapy; they do not do family therapy and they
are not able to supervise it; it is only the other disciplines
that can supervise family therapy. In our program, we have four
disciplines that are involved in teaching and supervising.

DR. CHRIST

I was just wondering about the need to teach two languages.
Somehow, I sense a feeling of near hopelessness in terms of the
amount that we have to teach. I am wondering if that is really
what you intended? I tell you why I am asking that. One of the
things that struck me is that the process of trying to learn something ourselves might take many many years. When we are in the
process of trying to uncover something new and there are muddy
times during that period, we might try to teach it and it comes
out very complicated. Once it becomes somewhat more clarified, I
have often been amazed as to how much can be conveyed in a
relatively short period of time to new people. I am wondering
whether your experience would lead you to feel that what you have
been describing as a teaching of two languages is something that
you have been able to now do in relation to trainees in a period
of one or two years.

DR. MALONE

I did not mean to make it sound so discouraging. However,
any serious effort to integrate family therapy into the core
curriculum of a child psychiatry program or a dynamically oriented
adult residency program is going to place quite severe demands on
the residents and on the faculty. I do not see any reason that
this difficult and challenging task should be seen as near hopeless.

It is frustrating, but there is a certain excitement from it too.
Sometimes, you do get discouraged. I find it much easier to teach
residents this bi-lingual approach than many of my most senior
colleagues. I respect these colleagues a great deal, but they
have considerable resistance to it. They will not teach against
it. They will not say do not use family therapy, but they really
do not understand the bi-lingual approach and resist it. I
accept that they are good at what they do and they are not ready
to make this kind of change. They continue to be superb supervisors of play therapy, individual analytic psychotherapy, and
group therapy, although the group therapy people usually are more
receptive and responsive to the family approach.

     I do feel, though, it has to be seen as a very serious under-
taking and one that takes quite a bit of work and that you work
at all the time. The faculty are gaining in their skills and
their experience all the time. I do think that many of the papers
so far have had common features, and that we are talking about
similar and certainly related kinds of issues. But this is a
complex field about which there is still a lot to be learned and
we are constantly learning. So I see it as a serious challenge
but one that has a lot of excitement and satisfactions as well
as frustrations.

DR. GOTTLIEB

     In the light of experiential change, do you think you could
get your fine individual supervisors and play therapy supervisors
to directly observe or to come into the room?

DR. MALONE

     Some of them, no. You are right.

DR. GOTTLIEB

     We feel the pressure on our shoulders to justify that. I
would think one of your earlier remarks this morning, maybe now
is the time to put the weight on the other shoulder. They should
be observing play therapy.

DR. MALONE

     Yes.

DR. GOTTLIEB

     They should be coming into the room.

DR. MALONE

They should be demonstrating how they do play therapy themselves. It is a very good point and we have placed that pressure,
but, interestingly, the same few faculty members are resistant in
that area as well as to the family approach. I think that they
really are locked into rather traditional views of the nature of
the therapeutic process. But I agree with you. I think the
challenge should be placed there. And, I agree very much with
what Dr. Christ said earlier, that a director should challenge all
the components of a program. Although I do not feel that family
therapy is just one of a series of components, it is much more
important than that. It is much more fundamental. But one should
place the same demands on each area of training. How are you
going to strive for excellence in a program if you do not do that?

THE ROLE OF FAMILY THERAPY IN CHILD PSYCHIATRY TRAINING: WHY AND HOW

Lee Combrinck-Graham, M.D.

Philadelphia Child Guidance Clinic

Philadelphia, Pennsylvania

An unsophisticated observer might be very surprised to learn that the family is not the natural domain of child psychiatry. This same naif might wonder why leaders in the field of child psychiatry would gather to grapple with the problem of how to train future child psychiatrists in the area of family therapy, when the field of child psychiatry itself is well over fifty years old. But the apparent rift between psychiatry for children and family therapy pits theories and therapies against each other which, we would agree with our wondering observer, do seem to belong together. Our first task, here, is to examine this problem with a goal to understand how the differences have been maintained, and how they might be reconciled.

DEFINITION OF CHILD PSYCHIATRY

As a beginning, let us try to define our terms. What is child psychiatry? First it is a medical specialty. As physicians, child psychiatrists are interested in the psychobiological aspects of children's behavior and development, and in this area can make medical interventions. But beyond the actual practice of medicine, child psychiatry refers to the humanistic attitude of the physician, the investment in the worth and dignity of people. It refers to the physician's responsibility to his patients, to their families, and to others concerned with their care. And it refers to the physician's responsibility for consideration of ethical matters and for decisions which concern life, death, disease and the overall quality of life.

Child psychiatry refers to the practitioner's concern for

113

children in the developmental process. The child psychiatrist is
trained to be familiar with phase specific issues which are age-
referenced, and he can say with certainty that children will change
with the passage of time. He must learn to predict in what
direction these changes are likely to take place and what forces
will affect them, particularly, to support the most beneficial
direction of growth.

Child psychiatry concerns itself with the behavioral sciences
beyond the realm of medicine. The child psychiatrist must be
familiar with the environment in which development occurs, the
family, the school, the peer group, the society, and, he needs to
understand the importance of these institutions to the child and
their effects on children.

Child psychiatry, then, is the integration in one field of
medical practice, developmental psychology and the social sciences
with the goal of intervening in those situations where children
do or will suffer from emotional disorders which threaten their
opportunities for optimum development into comfortable, productive
adults.

DEFINITION OF FAMILY THERAPY

What is family therapy? It is a therapeutic approach based
on theory that behavior occurs in a context, and the psychological
make-up of people is shaped and maintained in a context. Context
refers to the climate of attitudes, expectations, and habitual
modes of interaction around an individual as well as to the others
in his environment. In a broad sense, we could look at the context
of the planet earth in the solar system. The earth's movements
are a function of its interaction with the sun and the orbits of
the other planets. From another star, however, we could see the
solar system as a whole, moving in a still larger context. Clearly,
families are members of societies, ethnic groups, parishes,
neighborhoods, work forces, extended families, and so on. The
family itself, then, is a subsystem of a larger context.

Family therapy is a contextual therapy, and the family
therapist holds in mind the larger context and other contexts
relevant to family members. But the family having defined itself
as such, has a distinct identity over time and may, therefore,
be the most manageable group for ecological intervention. Particularly for children, the family context is most significant for
shaping and maintaining behavior, since children spend most of
their time and their most significant time in their families.
Family therapists concern themselves with the fact that individuals
resonate with their contexts and vice versa. In their practice,
family therapists use this knowledge as a basis for intervention.

If we accept these definitions--one of child psychiatry and the other of family therapy--we must realize that there can be no child psychiatry without consideration and involvement of the family. In the diagnosis of children who have difficulties of living, hindrances in development, impediments to age-appropriate task completion, is not the family context critical? And if this context is critical, can we really correct problems in the child without effecting some change in the family? We think not, and we think that child psychiatry has never been without thought to the family, and never can be.

CHILD PSYCHIATRY'S PROBLEM WITHOUT FAMILY THERAPY

What, then, are the problems--for problems there are? Some of the problems derive from traditional approaches to treatment which are conflicting about how and how much the family should be involved in the treatment of a child. An acquaintance of mine recently highlighted the issue of separation of child and family in treatment as a problem when she presented the following vignette. Her 9 year old son has been having school difficulties. He has been seen diagnostically by a psychologist and by a child psychiatrist. Serious concerns have been raised by the findings of these professionals who saw the boy alone. My friend, who did not witness the examination itself, is now being confounded by the grave predictions of the psychiatrist. A course of expensive and mysterious treatment is being proposed for ills which are now equally mysterious. My friend cannot expect the child's behavior to change for quite some time. She will be seen by an associate of the psychiatrist who will help her to adjust so as not to impede the boy's progress as he changes.

As a humanistic child psychiatrist, I have a few concerns about this procedure. My first is the lack of attention to the urgent need for relief of the boy's symptoms, made all the more urgent by his rapid development and his need to be flexible enough to pass from the issues of this phase to those of the next. A second is the egregious disrespect of the mother, an intelligent woman, who, having lived with her son for his whole life, no doubt knows him well. Now she must question her knowledge, and, even worse, must turn him over to someone outside the family who will see him a tiny percentage of his daily life. She might wonder if she is being blamed for causing his problems. But, at best, she must question her competence as a parent.

This model of practice is fairly prevalent in child psychiatry. It is a model which propounds that the child's problems are generated from within him, and this idea is derived from theories formulated from work with adults. It is a model which fails

to integrate consideration of the child in his context either
diagnostically or therapeutically.

CHILD PSYCHIATRY'S PROBLEM WITH FAMILY THERAPY

There are arguments on the other side. A particularly
articulate statement of problems for child psychiatry presented by
family therapy is made by McDermott and Char (1974). They crystal-
lize their presentation of the difficulties in three "myths" which
they attribute to family therapy's effect on psychiatric services
to children. Briefly stated they are: One, that the child is a
thermometer of family (marital) tensions; two, that a generic goal
of family therapy is communication and intimacy as well as autonomy
and individuation for its members; and, three, that the generalist
can be trained in family therapy techniques which, if one and two
are correct, leads to a diminished need for practitioners skilled
with children. In short, the concern expressed by McDermott and
Char is that the focus of family therapy will be away from the
child, and the child's special needs which are the concern of the
child psychiatrist will be overlooked altogether.

There is some validity to their concerns if one considers the
views of some of the leading family therapists. Virginia Satir
(1967) seems to reduce the causes of family dysfunction to
insecurities in the marriage. She also is a proponent of the
notion that good communication makes healthy people. Nagy and
Speck (1973) present the theoretical position that the expression
of pathology in an individual (a child, for example) is transmitted
through generations of loyalties and obligations within families,
so that the treatment involves a reworking of these complex
relationships through the past--a painstaking and time-consuming
process that often excludes the children.   Bowen (1976), too,
quickly moves from the troubled child to the dysfunctional couple--
his parents--who are "triangling" him in their own struggles with
each other for differentiation of self. And with Bowen, too, the
problem is seen to stem from family roots, so that the therapy
can be altogether removed from the child. These advocates of
family therapy do come from a background in adult psychotherapy,
so it is understandable that their attention to the specific
issues of children is less than satisfactory. However, if their
approaches are stretched to include families in which children are
the primary patients, then McDermott and Char have legitimate
concerns about family therapy.

CONTRIBUTION OF FAMILY THERAPY

There are approaches to family treatment which consider that

the child is developing in a family context with intervention
strategies designed to produce change in people, including and
especially children. It is approaches like these which must be
developed and refined to include the following components so that
they can be taught to child psychiatrists: Most suitable for child
psychiatry is an approach which considers the nuclear family of the
child in terms of its present functioning and the appropriateness
of its functioning for the developmental needs of its members.
Desirable, too, is the view that parents are responsible for their
children so that the hierarchal structure of the nuclear family
is supported. Attention must be directed to the urgency of
correcting dysfunctions in children because of their inexorable
movement through developmental stages. Erikson (1963) notes that
it is disadvantageous to drag one stage's unresolved issues into
the next. A relevant family therapy approach needs to deal
relevantly with current developmental issues and environmental
ones at the same time.

    A school of family theory and therapy which lends itself
especially to the treatment of children has come to be known as
"structural family therapy," which was introduced by Minuchin
(1974) and refined further by Minuchin, Rosman, and Baker (1977).
Since Minuchin is a child psychiatrist, it is not surprising that
his family therapy approach particularly concerns itself with the
nuclear family and its central functions of bearing, nurturing and
educating children. Structural family therapy integrates the
organization of the family unit and its subunits in such a way
that dysfunction of an individual family member is seen as a
projection of the failure of desirable interpersonal structures in
the family. All family members living in a household or closely
involved with one another, are included in the diagnostic process.
This approach looks at symptomatic behavior as it evolves from
interpersonal sequences in the family, and understands the symptoms
in terms of function or dysfunction of the family's structures.

    Because of the dynamic interactional quality of the structural
model, the presenting problems cannot be attributed to one individual
or subsystem in the family, though each one brings something special
to the situation. A child, for example, cannot be seen as either
fully responsible for his deviance or as a victim of others'
abuse of power. Similarly, parents can neither be absolved from
responsibility or fully blamed for their children's troubles. And
since it is the system which is dysfunctional when one member is
symptomatic, all family members are involved in the diagnosis.
Diagnoses in a family model shift away from the unsatisfactory
labelling of children to descriptive statements of interactional
sequences which occur particularly around the symptomatic behavior.
And because the interactions are occurring in the present, there is
a current relevance of the diagnosis which is just right for
child psychiatry. For example, Minuchin (1977) describes "rigid

triads" in psychosomatic families which are patterns of parent-child
interaction, where the child is involved in parental conflict-
avoidance in one of three characteristic ways. One of these rigid
triads, the "detouring-protective" pattern, describes a sequence
whereby parents can avoid conflict by caring for a sick child, or
avoid recognizing marital conflict by arguing over the care of a
sick child. In such a way, the child becomes the focus, and the
child's symptom becomes the means of maintaining a conflict-
avoiding pattern which in turn maintains the child's symptom. In
this case, the description of the dysfunction suggests therapeutic
action. In the case of the detouring-protective system, for
example, the therapist must stop the parents from arguing through
their child. They will be encouraged to express their disagreements
directly with each other and to resolve them, on the one hand,
and, on the other, to provide care for their child in such a way
that the child is differentiated from the parents.

There is no doubt that such an approach to psychodiagnostics
and to psychotherapy with children requires some major adjustments
in ways children are traditionally viewed by child psychiatrists.
Fundamental issues are raised: What about the intrapsychic life
of the child? What about the psychic structures that have already
formed? What place do these have in the family model? And, how
are they addressed in the treatment?

The answers are important theoretically. It appears that
intrapsychic representations in children, though they undoubtedly
exist, are, in fact, maintained in the context, usually that of
the family, and they seem to need some persistent reinforcement to
maintain them. This is not a new notion, nor is it exclusive for
family therapy. It has long been the basis of residential
treatment for children; change the context, take the child away
from the family, and then the pathological processes within the
child can change. Family therapy takes advantage of this
experience but in a more immediate way which is more crucial to
the needs of children. For example, a youngster who suffered a
head injury in an automobile accident was regarded as severely
handicapped and attended special school. Subsequently, she
perceived herself as extremely impaired, since she despaired of
being able to master academic subjects and did not know what she
could do. In the family, one could see the maintenance of this
self-view when other family members kindly supplied words when the
youngster halted and "reminded" her where they were when her memory
"lapsed" in the middle of a conversation (usually an argument).
Restraining the family members from this "helpfulness" created a
silence in these instances, which forced the child to find lost
words for herself and allowed her and the rest of the family to
experience her as more competent. The child did have learning
disabilities, but she had reached a plateau in her rehabilitation
which was unwittingly reinforced by the family interaction. After

the treatment, she was able to tackle learning situations with renewed energy, confidence, and skill and found herself to be more competent than she had thought.

What about those symptoms of "mental disturbance" which have always been regarded to reside within the patient? What about autism, psychosis, MBD? Are these thought to be caused by the family? We do not think that families cause accidents or produce biological damage. We could not even argue that families cause schizophrenia, the nature-nurture controversy being unresolved (Laing, 1965). The universal explanation is not to be found in family theory, nor is family therapy the universal cure. But at the time a family is being seen because of the difficulties of one of its members, it is likely that the family group has settled into some habitual patterns of interaction around the problem area which stabilizes it, and may exacerbate it, as in the example cited above.

For example, families typically treat the psychotic adolescent as incompetent, and, therefore, he is not expected to care for himself. Families often expect their "out-of-control" hyperactive youngster to be out of control and, therefore, don't intervene to control the child. Though there may be driving factors within the child or outside the family system, as in the case of group delinquent problems, the family's response often supports the continuation of symptomatic behavior rather than interfering with it. How often, for example, is the starving anorectic girl seen arguing with her parents about whether she is too fat while her food goes uneaten? In such cases the family is diverted from the critical issue (the child's survival through adequate nutrition) to an immediately irrelevant issue (the child's appearance), and in being so diverted further endanger their child. Many more examples can be brought to bear on this point. The context reflects the intrapsychic life of the individual and vice versa, but that the reflection in context among people is more visible and accessible to change, and, therefore, diagnostic and therapeutic efforts in this direction may be preferable.

TRAINING PROGRAM FOR CHILD FELLOWS

In the actual training of child psychiatrists, we encounter the challenge of working with young professionals, all of whom have come to child psychiatry with backgrounds in adult psychiatry. Typically, the previous training has been focused on the individual adult, using a medical model which stresses pathology in the individual. Even when child fellows come with some experience in family therapy, often this has been a form of individual therapy in a family group or group therapy, in which members of the group

happen also to be members of the family. We are faced with the
task of enlarging the young clinician's viewpoints in three areas:
the world of children, whose point of view is different from that
of adults; a developmental viewpoint which looks at changes with
time; and an ecological viewpoint which looks at behavior in
context.

The background of the trainee is important. Occasionally,
for example, we have had the opportunity to train pediatricians.
Unlike psychiatric trainees, they come with a background which has
been focused on the child. Because nearly all of the pediatrician's
patients are brought by parents to the doctor, it is second nature
to the pediatrician to think of the parent-child interaction as
part of his assessment of the patient. The background of the
trainee is part of his context, and the training approach has to
consider this in mounting an effective training effort.

The philosophy of our training program at the Philadelphia
Child Guidance Clinic is that the child's world and development
must be learned about in the context of the family, the school,
the hospital, and the institution in which fellows work and
children are seen. Our training program does not regard family
therapy strictly as a modality of treatment, but as the most
relevant approach to diagnosis and treatment of problems in childhood. Modalities of treatment may include individual, group,
family group, behavior modification, hospital-milieu, and pharma-
cology. But with an ecological point of view, each modality is
selected with a consideration of how this will be an intervention
in the child's context.

The trainee is required to think, on the one hand, of the
impact on the family of whatever treatment is selected. For
example, the decision to hospitalize a child often has the effect
of declaring the child's parents incompetent so that when the
child is discharged, the family may be less able to care for him
than before. On the other hand, the trainee is taught to be
aware of this effect on the system so that he can press for change
rather than maintaining sameness. A beginning trainee saw a
psychotic adolescent with his family. Responding to the habit of
taking care of the patient, he quickly was drawn in to manage the
patient's behavior in the session while the family members sat
around and waited. A contextually-oriented therapist would have
the same concern about the boy's symptoms, but would have asked
the family members to get the boy under control. In this way,
the family's presentation of illness in the youngster is challenged
and responsibility for the noxious behavior is placed back with
the family.

STAGES IN TRAINING

Taking advantage of our observations about the pediatrician's approach to the family context, we begin the training program by having the trainee assess a lot of children. In this way, his viewpoint shifts to the world of children, drawing upon the diagnostic and interviewing skills already acquired with individual patients. Beginning here, the trainee must traverse three major stages in moving from his individual, medical approach, to a contextual approach in the diagnosis and treatment of children.

The first stage is the understanding of how problems in a youngster, which the fellow first formulates in terms of intra-psychic dynamics, can be reformulated in terms of intrafamilial dynamics. The fellow is asked to think, for example, of what kind of family system maintains an obsessive-compulsive child? How do the defenses of orderliness, obsessive organization, and rituals fit into a family context? For one such child, the fellow speculated that the family could either be highly controlling, in which case the child's symptoms could be seen as a parody of the family's style, or an unorganized group in which there is no predictability. In either case, the fellow predicted that there would be some conflict in the family about order. Having made a hypothesis about the family organization, the fellow sees the family. In the above case, there was an issue of order in the family, with parents disagreeing about almost everything pertaining to the schedule for the children, expectations for neatness, and, finally, what to do about their son's repetitive shoe-tying.

The second stage is a practical one. The fellow is now accustomed to think of how problems in children reflect the context, but he continues to describe the family members as individuals and attributes motivation to them as individuals. In other words, he has difficulty initially seeing the family members as a part of the system and appreciating the reciprocity in their activities vis-a-vis one another. This is not to say that people are not individuals or that they do not have motivation from within. But in the operation of therapy in the ecological model, it is the nature of interpersonal space and sequences of interactions between people which are the targets of the therapist's interventions. If he be accused of dehumanizing individuals, think, for a moment of the functional dehumanization that a surgeon must accomplish in order to replace a cardiac valve. The therapist must likewise be practical about the function of his work.

An example of the fellow at the second stage of training is the following description of a family in which the eleven year old boy had been referred for psychiatric consultation because he had a chronic worsening kidney problem due to a neurogenic bladder.

The boy was required by his medical regimen to urinate on schedule, since otherwise he had urinary retention and reflux. But he did not follow the schedule, and his kidneys were in danger. The family complained of their chronic disorganization and fighting, and all said they could not get the boy to hold to the schedule, and they were worried about his neglect causing his kidneys to fail. Typically, the parents had been given conflicting in- structions by the pediatricians, to supervise the boy closely and to let him be responsible for himself. The model had been that the illness was in the boy, and the parents should cure it. The trainee's initial assessment of the family was in terms of the individuals. The boy was immature and deriving some secondary gain from his condition. The father was ineffective and impotent, and the mother was central and demanding, but impossible to satisfy. This assessment is correct, but stated in terms of individuals rather than the family system, therefore, implying that all the family members are "ill." What might be better from the contextual viewpoint is to say that mother and son have a stable coalition excluding father, though father is kept involved by the medical problems and concern for the boy's health. However, whenever the father tries to enter the system to care for his son, he is blocked by either mother or son, or both telling him that he does not know how to care for the boy; and the boy continues not to be cared for since there is no agreement about how it should be done. This formulation has the advantage that it can be confirmed by observation of how family members do interact and that it points towards intervention. To reiterate, this description does not focus pathology on individuals but looks at dysfunctional sequences between them.

When the fellow is comfortable with the work of the first two stages, he can also reverse the process so that having seen the family interact, he can quickly describe the individual child's experience of the problem, how it is maintained for him, and how the child is likely to carry the problem into other settings outside the family.

In the final stage, the fellow needs to learn how to inter- vene in a systemic way. Returning for a moment to our solar system analogy of contexts, the therapist looks at the family as if from another star. He sizes up the complex of forces which organize the system and calculates how he can intervene to change the system, knowing well that one move will affect everything. From his position outside the system, he might see that a comet will come dangerously close to a planet. He may wish to intervene by merely moving or removing the comet to change the way the other bodies interact. On the other hand, if he enters the system using his own force, this too can cause re- arrangements of the bodies. When a therapist intervenes in a family system, he alters the field. Therefore, he enters thoughtfully and deliberately.

This is really a most difficult stage of the fellow's
development. In his clinical experience with individual patients,
the trainee has created the interpersonal field in which the
patients change. In working with families, the therapeutic field
is made more complex by the numbers of people and their already
existing patterns. Therefore, he must learn to restructure the
system without being sucked in to pre-existing patterns, and,
therefore, rendered ineffective. To do this, he must assess in
advance the possible effects of his entry.

In the example presented of the family with the youngster with
a kidney problem, the therapist can support the hierarchical
organization of the family by insisting that the parents join
together to care for their son, at the same time blocking mother
and son's attempts to band together to disqualify father. The
therapist can carry out this restructuring by entering in one
of several ways. He could sympathize with the mother's frustration
at not being able to help her son, urging her to enlist the
support of her husband. He could chastise the father for not
being more effective in his role, and force him to confront his
wife when she undermines his attempts to look after the boy. He
can take the boy's part, reflecting that the parents are so
confusing that he does not know what to do. There is also a
position in relation to the siblings he could take. Where the
therapist chooses to enter first depends on his assessment of
where the power in the system is, where the system is most likely
to respond, where he, the therapist, is likely to have the most
effect, and numerous other considerations. At some time during
the treatment, the therapist may have actually taken all of the
positions described.

The three stages of training, one to translate diagnoses of
individuals to systems, the second to describe families systemically
rather than as complexes of individuals, and the third to intervene
systemically, all continue throughout the two-year program.
What we have done here is to describe a sequence to introduce the
fellows to ecological concepts in such a way that clinical skills
acquired in his previous training can be utilized and expanded
upon.

SUMMARY

In this paper, we have shown why we think that child psychiatry and family therapy are natural partners, inextricably
involved with one another. As often practiced in the past, both
child psychiatry and family therapy have suffered from theories
and techniques thought to be useful for adults, applied to the

treatment of children. This has yielded awkward and not particularly effective approaches to children. Strangely enough, this has also led to the dichotomy that one group sees the child without the family, and the other group sees the family without the child. The child and the family merge if one approaches the situation through the child directly. Child and family become inseparable in considering what the difficulties are and how they may best be treated. Therefore, theories and practices need to predominate in child psychiatry which begin with the child. To understand the child and what ails him, one must understand where he lives and what is most urgent for his current stage of development and what is needed to maximize his genetic potential. Child psychiatrists must be trained this way to deal relevantly with children. and their difficulties. The future of child psychiatry, we believe, is in the family.

REFERENCES

Bowen, M. Theory and practice of psychotherapy. In P. Guerin (Ed.) Family Therapy, Theory and Practice. New York: Gardner Press, 1976

Boszormenyi-Nagy, I. and Spark, G. Invisible Loyalties. New York: Harper and Row, 1973.

Erikson, E. Childhood and Society. New York: Norton, 1963.

Laing, R. D. The Divided Self. London: Pelican, 1965.

McDermott, J. and Char, W. The undeclared war between child and family therapy. Journal of American Academy of Child Psychiatry, Vol. 13, Yale, 1974.

Minuchin, S. Families and Family Therapy. Cambridge, Mass.: Harvard, 1974.

Minuchin, S., Rosman, B., and Baker, L. Psychosomatic Families: Anorexia Nervosa in Context. Cambridge, Mass.:Harvard, 1977.

Satir, V. Conjoint Family Therapy. Palo Alto, Calif.:Science and Behavior Books, Inc. 1967.

WHY ARE INTRAPSYCHIC DYNAMIC ISSUES LEFT OUT OF THIS FAMILY THERAPY MODEL? DISCUSSION OF DR. COMBRINCK-GRAHAM'S PAPER

Frederick M. Ehrlich, M.D.

Tufts University School of Medicine

Boston, Massachusetts

Dr. Combrinck-Graham's paper makes a forceful presentation of the need to include family, child and environment in our thinking in child psychiatry and then demonstrates the power of structural family therapy in dealing with these three components.

She then describes her program for teaching this approach. It is apparent that much thought and energy have gone into this training program and that an atmosphere of vigorous interaction between trainees and teachers has been achieved. I found most interesting in her paper the progression which she describes through what she calls three processes. These are: first, learning how intrapsychic dynamics can be reformulated in terms of intra-familial dynamics; second, seeing family members as part of a dynamic system; and, third, learning to treat the family system. I would be interested in hearing more about the progression through the three stages and how this is documented and monitored. I have found the assessment of the progress of a trainee to be a difficult matter.

There is, however, a theme in this paper which troubles me both as a child psychiatrist and a psychoanalyst. That theme is an uneasiness with the individual and an attack on the treatment of individuals. The paper opens with a bad example and ends with a good example; the bad example is of individual treatment and the good example is of structural family therapy.

I am reminded of an old saying: "For example, isn't proof." The first example is not fair; it is a second-hand report from a friend, a notoriously poor source of data about treatment.

We are assured, without documentation, that this treatment will
ignore the need for urgent corrective action, disregard the mother
who can then hardly escape blaming herself for her son's problems,
while the treatment pursues its leisurely if not obsessive examination of the boy. We are told that this valueless approach is
unfortunately all too common.

That poor treatment occurs I am well aware, but I must assert
that with my own eyes I have seen children in individual treatment
who have surmounted urgent problems and parents whose guilt has
subsided and whose self-esteem has flourished.

In the second example which describes a supervisor helping
a trainee with a family interview, we are told: "The prognosis
for psychosis in adolescents is not good. But the prognosis for
this girl is good because the doctor...brought to bear on the
case his concern, his understanding of developmental issues, and
his confidence in the healing processes within the family."

I, too, am impressed with the power of an accurate intervention but I would be loathe to suggest to a trainee that his
concern, understanding, and confidence had changed the prognosis
for a psychotic girl in a single intervention. I think people
are more difficult to change than that. This brings me to what
I sense as an underlying theme in this paper: an uneasiness with
the individual. Although individuals and their dynamics are
mentioned, it is as if they were distant relatives in the parlor
and the family is waiting for them to go away so it can get on
with its more intimate business. For example: "Intrapsychic
representations in children, undoubtedly exist, but are in fact
maintained in the context usually of the family and they seem to
need some persistent reinforcement to maintain them." Or again:
"This is not to say that people are not individual or that they
don't have motivation from within."

Why this tentativeness about inner structure and its
importance? Let me appeal to a different source to remind us how
important our inner structures are and how difficult they are to
know and to describe.

Robert Frost in his poem "Desert Places" describes the
loneliness of fields and woods covered with snow and then concludes:

> And lonely as it is that loneliness
> Will be more lonely ere it will be less-
> A blanker whiteness of benighted snow
> With no expression, nothing to express.

They cannot scare me with their empty spaces
Between stars-on stars where no human race is.
I have it in me so much nearer home
To scare myself with my own desert places.

Whether in the family or out, we carry our own inner world
including our desert places within us. Although we are altered
by our surroundings and the people with whom we interact, there
is something in each individual which is enduring and his own.
And so, in that sense, I find myself among the integrators who
feel we need both sides.

ARE THE ISOLATED FAMILY THERAPISTS SURROUNDED BY THE WOLVES OF

INDIVIDUAL THINKING? GENERAL DISCUSSION

DR. CHRIST

What are the integrative and nonintegrative aspects? What is lost and what is not lost in one approach versus another approach? I suspect that this will be probably one of the central areas of what we will be emphasizing in our ongoing discussions.

DR. GRUNEBAUM

First of all I sense that many of us speak specifically from the context in which we work. Are we the lone family therapist surrounded by the wolves of individual thinking? Or are we a family therapist surrounded by family therapists? It seems to me, however, that we should take sides. The individual therapists do not need advocates. In fact, in the battle on this issue of whether behavior is inherent in an individual or inherent in a context, it seems to me that at this point it may be useful to take sides. And the side we should take is the side that it is inherent in context. And I say this in part because we have talked a lot about this conflict as though it were located largely in psychiatry. It is not. This is a country where the rights of individuals are a theme of our history and where responsibilities between people are much neglected.

We are also in a capitalist system and are operating in a profession which is the last one of the strongholds of the entrepreneur. It is no wonder that individual thinking is much more compatible with the people with whom we work and the people with whom we teach, and they come to us from this context. Public health, preventive medicine, and other ecological and contextual approaches have never been very important in medicine. It seems to me we would look beyond the psychoanalysis and family therapy context to the broader context in which we are teaching. And I also think we should take sides.

DR. GOTTLIEB

I am distressed with Dr. Ehrlich's critique of Dr. Graham's
paper. I do not know where, quite, to put my finger on it.
Without psychopathologizing, as I think he did, in claiming that
Dr. Graham was setting up a straw woman with that first example,
I would suggest that maybe Dr. Ehrlich set up a straw woman and
critiqued in a way that really did not pay adequate attention to
Dr. Graham's data. I find my friends' stories about their
experience with psychiatrists very accurate, and I would subscribe
to the daily reality she described. Dr. Graham made a point
which really deserves an answer and discussion by Dr. Ehrlich
with his particular skills and interests. She said that a child's
intrapsychic life is maintained by the child's context and I would
think that this discussant might address that issue to better
inform us how he thinks a child's intrapsychic life is maintained.

DR. BROWN

I would like to return to the theme of integration because
I think it suddenly became a shadowy member of the community
here. If I can remind the group of the philosopher Hegel's
formulation: thesis, antithesis, and synthesis. I am reluctant
to say that Marx also used that formulation because that might
disrupt some people's equilibrium! The notion of integration
does not mean simply bouncing from one side to the other side and
hitting something halfway between. The notion of integration
means understanding that what presents as thesis eventually
becomes expressed or explored in an antithesis. The synthesis is
a re-combination in a dynamic sense, essentially a transformation
into a new level of knowledge and associated function. I think
if we keep that in mind, we do not get so worried about who is
on which side of the fence. What stays in mind is how each point
of view finds a certain reflection of its own truth in the other
point of view. The mental task therefore is to focus on the
continuing and unending process. The realization is that there
is not simply a final integration which will end the story, but
rather an endless process of thesis, antithesis and an integration
which then becomes the new thesis and so on. I am not a
professor of philosophy and I do not want to begin to sound like
one. But I do think that in debates, we lose track of that level
of understanding and an emotional polarization occurs within a
field as it has occurred in family therapy. I wish we could
put more creative energy into understanding the truth in each of
the sides and the back and forth interplay. So a little bit of
moralising from my side.

DR. CHRIST

Thank you Dr. Brown. It is an important issue, one that

I hope we will pick up on because the whole question does sound
a little bit too simplistic to merely say let us just synthesize!
A very dynamic process has to take place in which the various
aspects somehow in combination yields something new.

AUDIENCE MEMBER

I want to comment that we have to take sides. We need to
have data to work with and I do not think that neither the
individual proponents, nor the group and family proponents really
have the data to demonstrate one or the other has the right
answer. In my part of the country, we take a very pragmatic
approach.

DR. COMBRINCK-GRAHAM

I just love this. This is exactly what I hoped would
happen. I absolutely agree with Dr. Grunebaum that before we
reach the synthesis referred to by Dr. Brown, we have to take
sides. I am delighted by your comments. I am also delighted by
all those of you who came to rescue the one maiden here in
distress.

COMPREHENSION OF THE DEVELOPMENTAL CYCLE OF FAMILIES IN THE

TRAINING OF CHILD PSYCHIATRY CLINICIANS

Saul L. Brown, M.D.

Cedars-Sinai Medical Center

Los Angeles, California

INTRODUCTION

Learning to do effective clinical work with families is a
process that evolves slowly. It requires much more than the
initial enthusiasm that may follow a few successfully managed and
lively family interviews. Some early experiences of that kind
are essential for developing a belief in the value of the
modality, but the ability to hang in with difficult families over
a period of time requires a considerable depth of clinical wisdom.
That kind of wisdom about families accumulates slowly and builds
out of a combination of substantial theoretical comprehension and
wide ranging clinical experience including trial and error,
success and failure.

I will attempt to show the importance of the developmental
cycle as a theoretical framework for trainees. My conviction is
that an in-depth comprehension of development, in other words, an
historical orientation, is essential for stable and wise clinical
work with individual psychotherapy as well as with family therapy.
This does not mean, however, that history is used in every
clinical situation. It is well recognized that while comprehension of personality development provides a guide for a
clinician's work in individual psychotherapy, it may not influence
each case directly. The same is true for therapy of families.
My hope is that when trainees establish a genuine comprehension
of how families develop, decisions about the following will fall
into a stable frame of reference. What to focus on now? What
to avoid? What to postpone? What to seek auxilliary help for?
In this way, I seek to evoke the interest of those who do the
training, as well as those who are in training, to study seriously

133

the subtleties of family development.

The concern of this symposium with training of child
psychiatrists may seem to limit the following formulations more
than I would like them to be since, in fact, most family therapy
currently is being done by many excellent clinicians who are not
trained child psychiatrists. However, my personal identification
with the field of child psychiatry causes me to moralize that
unless child psychiatrists "get with it," they will lose the
opportunity to bring their highly developed skills and knowledge
into the field of family therapy and, thereby, influence those
who practice it. In my present work as the Director of a
Community Mental Health Center in the Department of Psychiatry in
a large medical center, I am in daily contact with the full range
of general psychiatric practice. I observe how much a background
in child psychiatry can contribute to effective work in general
psychiatry as well as in psychodynamic psychotherapy. I see, too,
how it might contribute to the work family therapists do.
However for this to occur, child psychiatry trainees must begin
to learn family therapy. With all that needs to be mastered during
child psychiatric training, two years of fellowship can be a
beginning only.

SOME EDUCATIONAL GOALS

From a family therapist's viewpoint, educational goals for
clinicians in the field of child psychiatry are at least the
following:

1. To establish a high degree of conviction that interviews
with an entire family group are of value

> (a) for the designated patient
> (b) for the parents of the patient
> (c) for the siblings of the patient
> (d) for the clinician and for all other professionals
>   who may be involved in providing help to the
>   designated patient.

2. To help the clinician achieve some facility with the
technique of interviewing family groups, even when family
therapy is not intended as the primary modality.

3. To provide clinicians who work with young patients a
theoretical frame of reference which gives purpose and direction
to the flexible use of family interviews and family therapy.

My task here is to contribute to the third educational goal,
namely to help establish a useful frame of reference that fulfills

an integrative approach to the work with families. I hope to
show how the training experience of the child psychiatrist can
be bent toward achieving that particular integrative capability,
if an understanding of the developmental cycle of families is
strongly emphasized.

SOME ANTECEDENT ASSUMPTIONS

     The following assumptions are essentially subjective and
reflect my experiences with beginning trainees and with many
experienced clinicians in child psychiatry. My purpose in
stating them is to help clarify and shape the educational problem
we are confronting in this symposium by first surveying the
characteristics of those we hope to train:

     A first assumption. Most individuals seeking training in
child psychiatry carry an old identification with the "hurt
child" and sometimes the "deprived child" which is relatively
unconscious or at least unformulated. Coupled with that
identification is a strong tendency to feel blameful of or judgemental of parents. Blameful attitudes toward parents are rarely
acknowledged, and even when acknowledged are usually accompanied
by an immediate effort to minimize their presence. Nevertheless,
as I have listened to students of child psychiatry discuss cases,
or sat with them as they observe family interviews on video tape
or through a viewing window, I have heard many spontaneous
comments and reactions from them that reveal barely contained
anger at the irrationality and the overt behavior of parents.
Short of undergoing psychoanalysis and becoming freed of old
antagonisms toward their own parents, how can trainees be lead to
a more positive feeling for parents of troubled children? My
hope is that an understanding of how a family system evolves may
help the trainee to avoid becoming locked into a persecutor and
victim view of parents and children. When one studies how an
interpersonal process unfolds, there is less inclination to be
judgemental and to over-identify with a single participant in the
process.

     A second assumption. For beginning child psychiatric
trainees, formulating the dynamics of a case may become a vehicle
for distancing from subjectively identifying with the day by
day phenomenology and emotional experience of life as it is lived
in the patient's family. I have observed this distancing most
regularly in medically trained psychiatrists and in academically
trained clinical psychologists, and somewhat less often in
clinical social work trainees and in some educational therapists.
Thus, while comprehension of individual dynamics and knowledge of
theories of behavior and of cognition are essential for intelligent
clinical work with children, they may be prematurely emphasized.

Intellectual formulations, even when correct, can too quickly close down an open sensitivity to the flow of emotions in a family. The result may be clinical methodology and case management that fails to keep in mind how the several family members of a family are affected by the behavior and problems of the designated patient. While learning about the developmental cycles of families does not always guarantee against such premature closure, it can challenge trainees to be alert to the roots of reciprocal feelings in all the familial relationships. Hopefully this loosens his/her over-reliance upon linear psychodynamic formulations and provides a greater openness to experiencing simply the family.

A third assumption. Many beginning child psychiatrists are quite unknowing about the nature of reciprocal process in multi-personal social systems. Except for those few who may have had earlier experience in social or business organizations, knowledge of such phenomena tends to be theoretical. Usually the trainee's personal model for group process is based upon what occurred in his or her own family, coupled with the years of growing up in the relatively authoritarian systems usually found in public schools and in medical schools. Since process in such systems tend to be syntonic with, and even reinforcing of the authoritarian role of "the doctor," the child psychiatry fellow may be only vaguely aware of how much that permeates his view of professional functions. Moreover, doctors traditionally have had the luxury of remaining somewhat aloof from the minutiae of interpersonal process that surrounds the implementation of medical care. Having written his orders, the doctor goes on his way while nurses and administrators are expected to go into action. Thus, for the trainee in child psychiatry, there may be much to undo and much to learn if he is to become disengaged from an internalized model of authoritarian dyadic relating between doctor and patient or parent and child. Through studying the evolution of behaviors and roles in families, the trainee may achieve deeper comprehension of how authority and power are exercised, roles are defined, action toward goals is implemented, interpersonal conflicts resolved, and communication facilitated within the family system. All of this constitute the relatively invisible process that shapes both normal and pathologic personal development. Such comprehension is much more encompassing than the notions of linear causality which reflect relatively authoritarian models that are common in employment relationships, as well as in the conventional teaching of etiology as it tends to be presented in many educational programs.

A fourth assumption. Most child psychiatry trainees are relatively young and are not likely themselves to have progressed much beyond the very earliest phase of parenthood. Indeed, many are not even married when they begin training. They may

not have yet experienced the existential complexities of marital
commitment which include relating to in-laws and fulfilling
sometimes unwelcome caretaking responsibilities toward another
person. They have not yet been awakened in the night by an
infant, or needed to postpone personal pleasures because of a
child's illness, nor needed to delay career gratifications because
plans had to be made for the childrens' activities. They may be
a long distance from the subjective experience of conflict with
spouse about the other's mode of relating to the children; and may
be quite unknowing of a parents' feelings of envy or competitiveness
in relation to a friend's or a brother's or sister's child. The
emotions of rage or disappointment or guilt over perceived
deficits in one's own child are still foreign to them. In other
words, the trainee may not have had much subjective contact with
the "stresses" of parenting. Once again, I hold some hope that
a deep knowledge gained during training of how family systems
develop can compensate for what the trainee has not experienced
and in that way create greater wisdom about how parents and
children affect one another.

      A final assumption. I believe many, if not most beginning
child therapists have somewhat romantic and exaggerated expectations
of what they can accomplish through conventional child therapy
techniques. Because such expectations often fail fulfillment,
there is a rapid turning away from doing child therapy by many
who have been trained in the field. These kinds of expectations
have, at times, become a belief system which assumes that appropriately formulated dynamic interpretations made to a troubled
child are enough to dissolve a child's problems. The necessity
for concurrent dynamic effort with the parents has often been
felt as a burdensome ancillary activity hopefully to be undertaken by others, (presumably social workers or educators). What
may have contributed to this belief system are the dramatic, even
exciting analytic case descriptions of the treatment of children
that have accumulated in the literature over the years. A
trainee may become focused upon replicating those clinical
experiences and may fail to develop a broad clinical frame of
reference and methodology for doing useful and gratifying work
with the large numbers of children who do not respond in finite
and crystal clear fashion to psychodynamic interpretation or
to play therapy. Once again, comprehension of the developmental
cycle of families can contribute to a more realistic view of the
factors affecting a child's pathology and a greater insight into
what may be necessary in order for therapeutic change to occur.

      Trainees must thread their way through the above in order
to reach the level of clinical wisdom we who have worked with
family therapy hold forth for them. In order to facilitate this
educational process, I believe that comprehension of developmental phases in the family life cycle is essential. However,

achieving such comprehension is much more difficult than may
appear at first glance. It involves more than a simple learning
of the developmental stages through which a family progresses.
While allusions often are made to the notion of developmental
phases in family life, relatively little has been written that
specifically integrates that particular kind of historical
emphasis with the here-and-now dynamics of family life. There
are, however, some significant contributions. Among them are
writings by Hill and Hansen (1960), Rapoport (1965), Solomon
(1973), Stierlin (1974), and Brown (1969, 1973). Notable for its
absence are contributions from established child psychiatrists
who have been intimately devoted to themes of family dynamics for
at least 30 years! A discussion of this disparity is presented
in a series of articles in the <u>Journal of the Academy of Child
Psychiatry</u>, (Vol. 13, #1, 1979), especially the one by Malone
/197<u>9</u>/).

SYSTEMS THEORY

A brief excursion through relevant aspects of interpersonal
systems theory will add an essential dimension to the historical
frame of reference which is my own primary emphasis in this
presentation. The concepts and language of systems theory
applied to families are necessary for effective clinical work with
children and families. Transactional role theory, an early
antecedent of systems theory as it relates to family process, has
contributed useful conceptual terms for understanding who does
what and how in families. The writings of Talcott Parsons (1955),
John Speigel (1971, and Nathan Ackerman (1958) all served to
enlighten us about how role functions are defined and how an
understanding of this deepens clinical insight. Moving forward
from role theory into systems theory has been a particular
contribution from clinicians such as Donald Jackson (1959), Jay
Haley (1963), Murray Bowen (1966) and Salvadore Minuchin (1969,
1974) to mention just a few. The work of Minuchin (1967, 1974)
has been especially useful for those treating children and
adolescents. Through clarifying how sub-systems in families are
structured and how that structuring affects the early childhood
experience in families, Minuchin has made an indelible contribution
to our understanding of family system pathology as it relates to
the emergence of clinical syndromes and symptoms in children.
Minuchin's (1967, 1974) writings are basic reading for any trainee
in child psychiatry. The following summary comments about systems
functions in young families have been developed by Minuchin in a
chapter entitled "A Family in Formation" in his book, <u>Families
and Family Therapy</u> (1974). There is value for trainees in placing
more emphasis upon the family development theme than Minuchin
tends to do. Such an emphasis stimulates commitment in the

trainee to understanding how historical factors determine the
resistance to change that the clinician is likely to encounter.
In other words, the more deeply we comprehend how change occurs,
both historically and in the here-and-now, the greater our
clinical wisdom about the resistance to change; and what we can
and cannot do about it.

Some years ago, largely prompted by my daily contact with
the therapeutic nursery school in our Department of Family and
Child Psychiatry, I begin to develop some working schemata for
what I viewed as a developmental cycle of families, particularly
emphasizing the resistance to developmental change in families.
I used Erickson's (1964) formulations of epigenetic psychosocial
developmental phases as a theoretical model. This model emphasizes
the carry-over of behavioral modalities from a previous phase
into the next one, but modified into new behaviors in accordance
with the phase appropriate needs and maturational capabilities
of the new or current phase. This carry-over notion applies both
to what might be normal ego functions as well as pathological
ones. In a major sense, Erickson's formulations were derived
from basic psychoanalytic theory. His concepts converged in
many ways with those of another psychoanalytic student of children,
Rene Spitz (1965) who drew upon embryology and the evolution of
the fetus as a way of illustrating how traumata and/or deficits
in the developmental process affect subsequent development. The
psychoanalyst, Balint (1968), drew upon the geologic example of
faulting in the layers of the earth and their effect on the super-
structure to illustrate the same theme I am referring to, namely,
the carrying forward into the present of old and insufficiently
resolved deficits in the normal developmental process.

The following is my schematic representation of the historical
phases in every family:

DEVELOPMENTAL CYCLE OF FAMILIES

PHASE I: ESTABLISHING BASIC COMMITMENT TO THE MARRIAGE

The developmental task is to manage successfully a relative
disconnection from each of the families of origin and a re-ordering
of commitments to old friends, social activities, occupational
and professional involvements, etc.

PHASE II: CREATING SUB-SYSTEMS FOR MUTUAL NURTURANCE

The developmental task is to build upon the successes of
Phase I and to establish a warm and empathic care-taking relationship which is open to the arrival of a first child, who in turn
will contribute to the mutuality of positive feelings.

PHASE III: DEFINING EFFECTIVE INTERPERSONAL AND INTRAPERSONAL
             MECHANISMS FOR ENCOURAGEMENT OF EACH PERSON'S
             INDIVIDUALITY AND AUTONOMY

The developmental task is to draw upon the basic commitment
in the marital relationship and the nurturing spirit of the
young family evolved in Phases I and II, and through these to
provide spontaneous and warm encouragement of the personal growth
of each family member, in accordance with the levels of maturation
and the adaptive tasks each is confronting.

PHASE IV: FACILITATING EGO MASTERY FOR EACH FAMILY MEMBER

The developmental task is to draw upon the successes of
Phases I, II and III in order to provide family system competence
for helping each member to meet the ever proliferating existential
challenges that face each as he/she adapt to the world outside
the family as well as to the integrative stresses in individual
psychic development.

PHASE V: MAINTAINING FAMILY INTEGRATION DURING ADOLESCENCE
           AND YOUNG ADULTHOOD

The developmental task is to sustain integrated family life
through the various sub-systems that have evolved over the
previous years, even as the impact of adolescence challenges
family value and belief systems, the marital commitment, the
intergenerational boundaries, the communication patterns, the
alliances, the individual identities, the sexual adaptations,
etc. that characterize the family life.

PHASE VI: ACHIEVING MUTUAL VALIDATION

The developmental tasks of this phase are multiple involving
the reworking but continuing integration of family relationships
so as to preserve the capability of the family system to provide
validation of each member as a lovable and valued person.

Clearly, the phases as I have presented them reflect an
ideal. Debate about the likelihood of achieving them in family
life belongs elsewhere. However, in another context, I have used
them to argue the theme of "basic requirements for becoming
human." My belief is that until society is organized so that the
phases of family development can evolve well, the likelihood of
achieving human potential at both an individual and a societal
level is small.

What is of importance for clinicians is that the schemata
provide a framework for evaluating where a particular family
system is failing now as well as where it has failed in the past.

Guided in this way, a clinician has opportunity for directing
his/her efforts so they are useful and constructive for both
child and parents and are in accord with what the family system
can accept. Relating this to the theme of <u>resistance to change</u>,
the trainee can gain insight into how resistance to developmental
change in the family system converges with the resistance to
therapeutic change that may be occurring in a particular case
(Barnhill and Longo, 1978).

FAMILY SYSTEMS AND SUBSYSTEMS

     Having emphasized the historical dimension in the systems
view of families, I will briefly recapitulate those aspects of
family experience that may be characterized as subsystems. A
certain confusion quickly arises for the trainee in differentiating
the structural sub-systems in a family from the functional or
transactional sub-systems which is clarified by Minuchin (1974,
p. 51):

     "Family structure is the invisible set of functional
     demands that organizes the way in which family members
     interact. A family is a system that operates through
     transactional patterns. Repeated transactions es-
     tablish patterns of how, when, and to whom to relate,
     and these patterns underpin the system...Repeated
     operations in these terms constitute a transactional
     pattern."

Minuchin notes that individuals may be sub-systems within a family
as well as dyads (husband and wife or parent and child); and
each person belongs to more than one subsystem. Sub-systems may
be defined by generation, by sex, by interest or by function.

     Bringing together the historically oriented developmental
phases with the relatively more here-and-now oriented transactional sub-systems, one can conceive of the Developmental Phases
in a vertical axis and the transactional sub-systems on a
horizontal plane. The transactional sub-systems operate at all
times and exist, so to speak, within each developmental phase.
However, during a given phase in the history of a family, certain
sub-system transactions might have greater import than others.
For example, in Phase III, when individuation and autonomy are
major issues for the family, extremely clear and supportive
communication is a dominant issue. In Phase II, sharing affect
with all members, empathic relating and smoothly functional
sexual sub-systems may be primary transactional concerns that
overshadow others. Pervading each developmental phase are
transactions related to the resolution of interpersonal conflict.
Relative failures of function of this sub-system in any phase

erodes the function of all other sub-systems. Successful mastery
of each phase carries over into subsequent phases but relative
failure becomes a resistant to the normal progression of developmental change.

Overlapping and residing within each of the developmental
phases are the following transactional sub-systems that I find
useful to demonstrate to trainees. I ask them to think about
them relative to their own families:

The mutual nurturance sub-system--those processes,
emotional and physical, through which each person cares
for or is cared for by others.

The affectional sub-system--those interpersonal
patterns through which positive feelings are shown
and shared between all family members.

The empathic sub-system--those interpersonal
patterns that reflect each person's identification
with the feelings and experience of the other.

The sexual sub-system--the ways in which sensuality
is expressed and received.

The communication sub-system--the processes through
which feelings, ideas, views and needs are verbally
and explicitly stated or are nonverbally but clearly
expressed.

The autonomy sub-system--the mechanisms through
which each person achieves relative individuation
and separateness appropriate to age and family
structure, while still maintaining connection to
others; and the mechanisms through which each
person offers encouragement or discouragement to
the others.

The parental coalition and the intergenerational,
parent-child sub-system--the structural aspects
of the family--the alliances, how relationships
between generations are monitored, loyalties
encouraged, rules defined, feedback facilitated,
ties to older generation maintained. How parents
work together.

The conflict-resolution sub-system--overshadowing
and interwoven with all of the others, how
differences between family members are confronted,
how resolution occurs; presence of scapegoating,

depreciation, denial, projection, splitting,
etc.

<u>The pleasure-in-action sub-system</u>--the imple-
mentation of mutually gratifying experiences
for all family members and the completion of
goals and tasks.

The reason for delineating these sub-systems is the fact
that they constitute the substance and matrix of marriage and
family. They are in constant ebb and flow and in ever shifting
interface with each other. For medically trained residents,
an analogy to what one sees through an electron microscope may
be helpful. In contrast to the fixed cells of traditional
histology, we see a field containing constantly interacting
elements which, like DNA strands and intracellular bodies, interface, combine, change shape, split, recombine, and so on.

The dyadic process of Phase I of a family evolves over several
months, perhaps years. The form it takes reflects the mores and
rules of the socio-cultural tradition and environment in which a
couple live. Accordingly, the expectable marital behaviors in
a new marriage occurring in an authoritarian social environment
are very different from those expected in an egalitarian liberal
one. Even with a more liberal sub-culture, expected behavioral
patterns in the first phase of marriage may vary considerably.
Feminism has added even more complex variations to this them. My
main point here is that interpersonal behavioral patterns
established in the first phase of a family cycle need to fit well
with the immediate social environment of the couple. Even as
the commitment in the first phase forms, the couple should be
progressing into Phase II, namely the one of Mutual Nurturance.
Again, I emphasize that the interpersonal patterns and the
familial structure for providing mutual nurturance that develop
in Phase II need to be syntonic with the prevailing social
traditions and values of a particular couple. This is a most
important notion for trainees to grasp. Otherwise, the tendency
is for the clinician to try to guide a couple or a family according
to his or her own values, failing to perceive the subtle inter-
.actions in the family that affect its own sub-culture. The
family "Don" in the Italian mafia tradition is intensely
committed to his marriage, whatever his other social commitments
and activities may be like. Also, he nurtures his wife and
family according to his style and he receives nurturance from
them, according to the rules and patterns of that social sub-
system. How mutual nurturance occurs in such a social milieu may
offend the liberal values of a mental health clinician, but those
values need to be secondary to whether interpersonal transactions
in a given family are in fact facilitating the mutual nurturance
necessary in Phase II. If they are not effectively organized,

it is of some significance to decide whether the dysfunction
derives from and is a carry-over of developmental deficits in
Phase I or whether the observed familial dysfunction in Phase II
is simply a result of limited knowledge and of immaturity. In
the latter case, the failure to develop a mutually nurturing
environment when an infant arrives can be corrected through
providing education and guidance to the parents. In those cases
where dysfunction of mutual nurturance is largely a result of
failures to master Phase I, the major remedial efforts will need
to be directed toward helping the couple to reclarify their
marital commitment (keeping in mind the values and standards of
their particular social sub-culture). Again, clinical wisdom will
define whether marital counseling is needed or whether some form
of educational guidance will be enough for the couple to retrieve
what they failed to achieve in that earlier phase.

If the dysfunction of Phase II turns out to be deeply rooted
within the individual psychodynamics of the parents, an educational
or guidance approach related to Phase I and/or Phase II will not
be sufficient. While these might be components of early clinical
management, the positive changes one would hope to achieve for
successful mastering of Phase II may require a more intensive
therapeutic effort. That effort might be family therapy but
may also need to include individual therapy for either or both
parents and it may require play therapy or even a therapeutic
school for the child. In short, clinical management that is
based upon an understanding of how a family system develops are
more parsimonious and better focused than if the clinical management is dominated by an here-and-now orientation. The family
developmental orientation defines and may attend to earlier
developmental faults. Without remediation, the family system
may fail to sustain integrated function in its later and more
complex phases, despite the valiant efforts of individual therapy.

Illustration. In an early family interview with
four year old Marianne and her parents and her one
year old brother, Marianne was miserable. She clung
to her mother, would not come over to the attractive
play table around which we were all seated, and was
whiny and naggy and made constant efforts to poke
into or push at her mother's body. Her father did
not try to interrupt the fusion between mother and
Marianne. Mother provided Marianne with almost no
encouragement to relate to me or even to the toys
on the table.

In subsequent work with this family it became
evident that each parent had remained deeply attached
to their own parents. Neither felt emotionally safe

with the other. While on the surface they
appeared to be a fairly typical middle-class
young couple with the usual social adaptations
and skills, we learned that a major developmental
failure had occurred in Phase I of their family
cycle. The parents had not become genuinely
committed to the marriage. Subsequently, in
Phase II, while meeting minimum requirements of
mutual care-taking and nurturance, an under-the-
surface failure of empathic responsiveness between
the parents persisted as a developmental fault
in the family system. The absence of spontaneous
emotionally supportive gestures and comments between
the parents showed the failure to have mastered
Phase I and revealed the underlying fault which was
undermining the successful mastery of Phase II.
Moreover, the functional failures already pervading
Phase II had limited the family's capacity to
progress into and master Phase III, the one of
mastering individuation and autonomy. It is in
this phase that the emergence of individual
autonomy and the individuation of each family
member needs the support and nurturance that
ought to have become well structured and functional
in Phase II

To repeat an earlier point, in Phase I, sub-systems need to
evolve which establish role-functions that are mutually acceptable
to the married partners. In addition, communication processes
that are increasingly precise and well understood by the two
partners are essential if the marital bond is to "take." Effective
mechanisms for conflict resolution are necessary and they need to
incorporate concern for each other's well being. Along with
these sub-systems for shared feelings, sensuous needs and some
kind of sexuality should be evolving. Ideally, each of these
transactional sub-systems should be functional and reasonably
vital when the couple progresses into Phase II and by the time the
first child arrives. If, in Phase I they are indeed functional,
the mechanisms for providing mutual nurturance in Phase II are
well in place. The newly born family members quickly identify
with those mechanisms and add to them by virtue of the natural
spontaneity and warmth that infants bring. In this way, even the
infant nurtures the parents. The process of triadic relating
that occur around an infant become mutually enhancing under these
positive circumstances, rather than a source of strain and
confusion for the parents. Trainees can understand this best if
in taped interviews of families with very young children, these
issues are carefully reviewed, even while they may seem all too
"obvious."

Illustration 2. Even before Marianne's birth, her
parents repeatedly withdrew from one another and
turned to their own parents at times of conflict
with each other. An increasing emotional distance
created gaps in their communication with each
other. Feelings and thoughts could not be
verbalized in clear and anxiety reducing ways.
This was evident in the first family meeting.

Confusion occurs in young children when their parents are
unhappy with each other. Since clarifications for Marianne
rarely occurred, she became locked into primitive methods for
dealing with her own developmental stresses. Her behavior was
regressive. She clung to her mother but with ambivalence which
was intensified by the birth of her baby brother. She acted out
infantile fantasies of being held and fed, placing herself into
self-tormentive competition with her infant sibling and losing
opportunity to receive age-appropriate nurturance from adults.
Also she missed out on the experience of giving warmth and
positive feelings to others. She (and her parents) could not
become participants in the circularity of gratifying mutual
nurturance that should characterize Phase II and which becomes a
basis for mutual interpersonal relating in Phase III.

In Phase III, defining mechanisms for mutual encouragement
of individuation and autonomy are principal developmental tasks
of the family. These are in parallel with the individual
developmental tasks of the children who are toddlers or of pre-
school age in this phase of the family cycle. Trainees can become
conscious of how the process of individuation and movement
toward autonomy that characterizes this age is intertwined with
the development of facilitating mechanisms for the entire family
system. In this phase, each parent should also be defining
separate identities, but doing so in a mutually nurturing
fashion.

In conventional middle-class life, this individuation
process for the woman includes a growing competence to function
as a mother who must master the many complicated tasks of child
rearing, homemaking, socializing with neighbors, and maintaining
a network of friends. For many women, establishing a vocational
or professional career may also be occurring in this phase. For
the husband, the individuation process is one of becoming a
father and also it is usually closely tied to his development
in a professional or vocational field. As we well know the
conventional middle-class model does not apply universally.
However, I believe it is a social model that has value and is
worth striving for if it is radically modified by shared tasks
between the parents rather than rigidly defined sex-linked

functions. The main point is that in this phase, the parents must
be stabilizing their identities as relatively mature adults who
can provide leadership for their children. Doing this requires
that each support the other's individuation and all develop
effective social skills, with an ability to communicate feelings
and needs to one another in direct and clear fashion. In this
phase, the greatly expanded range of personal action requires even
more effective means for resolving conflicts, for planning
together, for implementing action, etc.

> Illustration 3. Mariann'e parents had become "stuck"
> and were not progressing successfully into Phase III.
> Their well entrenched tendency to withdraw from each
> other and to be defensive and distant rather than to
> clarify and resolve conflicts depleted their energy
> for collective family action around mutually pleasure-
> ful activities, and their ability to encourage progressive
> individuation in Marianne and in each other. They
> rarely made plans for family outings, and when they did,
> a spat between them or a temper tantrum on Marianne's
> part collapsed the effort before it began. Also,
> their regressive ties to their parents kept intruding.
> There were all too few times when the new family
> functioned in an integrated way, well separated from
> the grandparents (Failures from Phase I of the
> family cycle).

The relatively limited communication of positive feelings
in the family resulted in many unfinished discussions so that the
clarification of emotionally laden ideas as well as the transmission of information about surrounding interpersonal events and
phenomena were not occurring as they should. Curiosity and lively
exploration of ideas about people found new channels of encouragement in the family system during the developmental phase when each
parent might have been helping each other and providing models
for Marianne. Problem solving as a functional sub-system of
family life in Phase III was uneven and rarely capable of sustain-
ing mutuality of effort. Although each parent was individually
capable of complex activities in the external social environment,
they were unable to carry these out in joint efforts. Thus, the
failed nurturance of Phase II now become revealed in the lack of
warm spontaneous support for each person's individual growth. The
resistance to developmental change now operant in this small and
young family could be outlined and shown to represent the cumulative
failures in each developmental phase. For trainees, opportunity
to observe this progression through direct viewing of family
interviews and tapes opens comprehension of the complexity
inherent in a family approach to clinical problems. Also, it
helps to dilute the notion of individual victimization (of child
or of either parent) since the focus of the clinical intervention

is upon reducing the system's resistance to developmental change
rather than upon the malevolent effects of one or the other parent.
Resolving intrapsychic conflict in each parent or the child may
become necessary for the progress to occur, but clinical efforts
in this direction need to await clear delineation of how the
system functions and where the resistances to change lie. In a
case such as the one of Marianne's family, a sequence of clinical
efforts were introduced. Some were directly educational. Conjoint
therapy with the parents was tried but with modest success.
Marianne was seen individually in play therapy but only after
mother and she had been helped to give up the fusion with each
other through enrolling Marianne in our therapeutic nursery school.
She became able to achieve a substantial degree of individuation
but limitations in family functions were persistent.

TRAINING PROGRAM

     For the balance of my presentation, I will describe aspects
of the psychiatric training program at my institution and how family
therapy and development are integrated into the program.

Seminars

     During the second year, psychiatric residents meet in a one
year weekly seminar on Personality Development. This is essentially
a prelude to later training in child psychiatry for those who
choose it. In the Personality Theory Seminar, a psychodynamic-
psychoanalytic frame of reference is presented, but includes an
emphasis upon the transactional theories that derive from family
therapy. Video tapes of ongoing or recent cases which show family
meetings with toddlers and pre-school age children seen in the
toddler and pre-school centers of the Department are used for
illustration of themes. In summary, our educational objectives
are to:

     1. Review standard developmental theories of childhood
     2. Integrate psychoanalytic-psychodynamic theory with
         the transactional interpersonal theories
     3. Use video tapes to make more vivid how family
         transactions affect individual development and
         pathology in early childhood.

Observation

     Third year and other graduate level trainees observe a
family interview conducted by myself or by the Associate Director

of Family/Child Psychiatry at least once every two weeks. Alternatively, our Chief clinical psychologist or an experienced senior clinical social worker may do the interviewing. For the psychiatric residents, the question of role model and identity are significant and, therefore, it is important for a psychiatrist to do many of the family interviews. The trainee to whom a particular case is assigned is always present in the interview room.

Following the interview, observers discuss the clinical observations. Family developmental themes are often introduced in the discussion by the senior staff interviewer, thereby shifting content from a pure examination of communication mechanisms or current transactions. However, these discussions are spontaneous and an exact format is not adhered to.

The educational goals of observed interviews are:

1. To demonstrate not only the feasibility, but the singular value of family interviewing as a basis for clinical planning
2. To demonstrate how process occurs in family interviews especially as it relates to children
3. To clarify developmental themes evident in the family system
4. To teach family dynamics
5. To provide early professional role models for those trainees who are responsive to working with families.

Assignments

Third year Residents (and other trainees) are expected to include one or more family interviews in the evaluation process of each case assigned to them during rotation through the Family/Child Department. Child Fellows are assigned many more than this number.

The educational objectives are to:

1. Guide trainees toward a flexible model of clinical theory and practice
2. Show how family interviewing in the course of a case evaluation may be essential for realistic case management
3. To demonstrate that family interviews during the course of case evaluation does not always lead to using family therapy, but that developmental factors are significant for case management planning.

Child Fellows

     Ours is a division of Family and Child Psychiatry. Those
who choose to train with us usually have some notion that family
therapy is of major interest to our staff and frequently a
component of evaluation and case management process. In the
Child Fellowship, theory related to family systems is presented
alongside traditional theory. Family therapy literature review
is introduced early.

  1. During the first year of the child fellowship training,
     direct observation in the therapeutic pre-school centers
     and toddler center that are a part of our Department are
     required. For a part of the year, attendance at the
     weekly case conferences of those respective units is
     required. Because the children are very young, those
     conferences inevitably focus upon the development of
     pathology in the early phases of a family system. Many
     of the conferences include direct observations of family
     interviews done by senior staff. Opportunity is present
     to observe toddlers and pre-school age children in
     their sibling interactions as well as in interaction with
     parents.

  2. The value and conduct of play technique with very young
     children in family interviews is a major content of
     observed sessions.

  3. Concurrently, I do an observed weekly continuous case
     either with a child in age group 2 1/2 to 5 years, with
     the parents frequently present in some part of many of
     the sessions; or an observed continuous case with a family
     group that extends over a few months. Developmental
     tasks of the family system are easily demonstrated
     through these experiences.

Educational objectives are to:

  1. Demonstrate the value and feasibility of conceptualizing
     within both an individual developmental model and a
     transactional family model of therapy
  2. The senior staff instructor provides a role model for
     how a family therapist can combine an educative with a
     dynamic interpretive style of relating to a family
     when he/she comprehends family developmental theory.

DISCUSSION

     The training of psychiatrists in our Department includes a

continuous and ongoing experience with aspects of family theory and interviewing from at least the second year of training. The educational goal is to evoke an acceptance of the modality. A particular sub-goal of the training is to introduce the understanding of developmental sequence in family experience along with sensitivity to transactional tasks within each phase. The ultimate educational goal is to establish a point of view in the trainees that comprehends the reciprocity in one-to-one interpersonal relating and in group process that is cognizant of family system functions in the here-and-now and in their historical-developmental origin.

Needless to say, our educational goals are not always achieved. There is a high level of initial resistance in many trainees to meeting with a family group, especially when the children are very young. We observe in many trainees an almost palpable drift back toward one-to-one sessions in spite of all that has been described above. We assume additional experiential training is indicated to overcome this, but receptivity is essential and it may be limited to a minority of those who train in child psychiatry. Experiential training needs to include some role playing and simulated family therapy experience toward which child psychiatry trainees are not initially inclined.

SUMMARY

I have presented a somewhat over-condensed review of family developmental theory coupled with a rapid run-through of family systems theory placed against the backdrop of the developmental phases in a family cycle. My intention has been to show that this kind of double comprehension of family system theory plus family development theory provides an essential dimension in the educational process of child therapy clinicians. Implicit in my presentation is the notion that these concepts and insights can be taught to clinicians in training through the medium of family interviewing. Additionally, I have outlined some of the ways in which our training program functions.

REFERENCES

Ackerman, N. W. Psychodynamics of Family Life, Diagnosis and Treatment in Family Relationships. New York:Basis Books, 1978.

Balint, M. The Basic Fault: Therapeutic Aspects of Regression. London:Tavistock, 1968.

Barnhill, L. and Longo, D. Fixation and regression in the family life cycle. Family Process, Vol. 17, December, 1978, pp. 469-478.

Bowen, M. The use of family theory in clinical practice.
    Comprehensive Psychiatry, 4, 345-373, 1966.

Brown, S. L. Diagnosis, clinical management and family interviewing
    In: J. H. Massermen (Ed.) Science and Psychoanalysis,
    New York:Grune and Stratton, 14:188-198, 1969.

Brown, S. L. Family experience and change. In: R. Friedman (Ed.)
    Family Roots of School Learning and Behavior Disorders.
    Thomas, 1973.

Brown, S. L. and Reid, H. The warm line: A primary preventive
    service for parents of young children. In: H. Parad,
    H. L. P. Resnik, and L. G. Parad (Eds.) Emergency and Disaster
    Management, Bowie, Md.:Charles Press, 1976.

Erickson, E. Childhood and Society, (Revised Edition). New York:
    Norton, 1964.

Haley, J. Strategies of Psychotherapy. New York: Grune and
    Stratton, 1963.

Hill, R. and Hansen D. The identification of conceptual frameworks
    utilized in family study. Journal of Marriage and Family
    Living, 22:299-311, 1960.

Jackson, D. D. Family interaction, family homeostasis, and some
    implications for conjoint family psychotherapy. In
    J. Masserman (Ed.) Individual and Familial Dynamics. New
    York:Grune and Stratton, 1959.

Malone, C. Child psychiatry and family therapy: An overview.
    Journal of American Academy of Child Psychiatry, Winter, 1979,
    Vol. 18:1, pp. 4-21.

Minuchin, S., Montalvo, B., Guernez, B. G., Rosman, B. L., and
    Shumer, F. Families of the Slums: An Exploration of their
    Structure and Treatment. New York: Basic Books, 1967.

Minuchin, S. Families and Family Therapy. Cambridge:Harvard
    University Press, 1974.

Parsons, T. and Bales, R. F. Family, Socialization and Interaction
    Process. Alencoe, Illinois, Free Press, 1955.

Rapoport, R. Normal crises, family structure, and mental health.
    In: H. Parad (Ed.). Crisis Intervention. New York:
    Family Service Association, 1965.

Solomon, M. A developmental conceptual premise for family therapy.
    Family Process, 12:179-188, 1973.

Spiegel, J. Transactions (Edited Papers). Science House, New
    York, 1971.

Spitz, R. The First Year of Life. New York:International
    Universities Press, 1965.

Stierlin, H. Separating Parents and Adolescents. New York:
    Jason Aronson, 1974.

LUMPERS AND SPLITTERS: A PARADOX FOR PSYCHIATRY. DISCUSSION OF DR. BROWN'S PAPER

Lee Combrinck-Graham, M.D.

Philadelphia Child Guidance Clinic

Philadelphia, Pennsylvania

I was very much taken with Dr. Brown's characterization of the neophyte child psychiatry trainee and the typical unpreparedness of these trainees to work with children and families--not simply from the point of view of knowledge, but from that of experience.

I thought again of the characteristic depression that befalls our fellows in the first six months of training and of all the efforts we had made to reduce this by "making a transition" "building theoretical bridges" "emphasizing consistency with previous training," etc. The crisis in our fellows' lives appears to be precipitated by beginning child psychiatry training with an interpersonal focus at a new place. And I must say we have not been successful in eliminating it, or even reducing it significantly. As I thought about it some more, I decided that it was better that we had not eliminated it, for the affect we see is a response to the confrontation with new experiences, new ways of working with clinical material, and new theories. The affective response may be the disorganization which follows a crisis which is then followed by a heightened receptiveness to different ways of operating.

I then began to think about a paradox involving lumpers and splitters. It goes like this: There are two kinds of people in the world, those who believe that there are two kinds of people in the world and those who do not. Imagine the dilemma of those who do not when trying to ascertain which kind of people they are!

I began to wonder whether we do not create a similar dilemma when we say there are child psychiatrists and adult psychiatrists;

there are family-oriented psychiatrists and individually-oriented
psychiatrists; but all psychiatry is basically the same. And let
me complicate the picture further by asserting that in fact there
must be some fundamental similarities about all psychiatrists,
even if it be only that they all call themselves psychiatrists.

But what I would like to do, since I do believe that there
are at least two kinds of people and many kinds of psychiatrists,
is to focus on some differences.

First, I would like to talk about concepts of development--of
which there are certainly more than two kinds. One common notion
in development is that it is a kind of continuous epigenetic
process, with one stage being built on the accomplishments of the
previous ones. This is a very useful concept. But if one thinks
about the dismal failure we have had in attempting to predict an
outcome from the status of a person at a given point in time,
then one may instead be fascinated by episodes which may not even
be developmental, but which simply radically alter the course
of a person's life. One example is that of a 14 year old girl
who seemed bound to spend the next few years of her life in
institutions because of her failure to function. But then
something unexpected happened. Her mother died of a heart attack
in the courthouse while waiting for her daughter's case to be
heard. The girl joined her estranged family in planning the
mother's funeral, went to live with an aunt, and four years
later, has continued to progress in school without having entered
any institution. This outcome could not have been predicted. In
studying developement, then, it is important to have a sense of
the flow, but also understand the power of the unexpected to alter
this flow.

In looking at a developmental approach to families, another
kind of issue about similarities and differences arises--that
of stretching a theory developed for individuals to serve for
multiperson systems. One problem in doing this is that the
family developmental theory tends to favor some individuals in
the family. Dr. Brown's theory sounds as if it favors the adults.
A scheme that I have toyed with tends to focus on the children
as milbournes in the developmental life of the family. Each
falls short of a true systems theory probably because of the
procrustean efforts involved in adapting it from another genre.

Proceeding from this point, there are many problems in trying
to build a systems theory on psychological theories developed
for individuals. While individual psychodiagnostic theory is
very useful, I do not believe that it can or should be the basis
for studying and evaluating family systems. The descriptive
language is different, even changing for describing dyads and
triads. Many authors from diverse backgrounds have emphasized,

for example, that the dynamics of a dyad--such as a couple, or a
patient-therapist dyad are dramatically different from that of a
group of three or more. For example, the language of dyads
includes the words "symmetry" and "complementarity." While the
language of triads includes "triangulation," "detouring," "go-
between," "stabilizing." It appears to be impossible to capture
the group with the language developed for one or two. One is a
linear language, the other circular. Multiperson systems tend
to be circular, it not being possible to be certain where an
action really begins, while one or two person systems are linear
and can be described in cause and effect terms.

Finally, the study of the child, himself, defies real
continuity with the study of adults. The child's personality, for
example, cannot be descriptively crystallized, being in formation
and flux. Even temperament, advertized as a stable characteristic
of children, is manifestly different at different stages of the
child's life. As an object for study himself, the child with his
disarming frankness, his indirectness, and his use of the primary
process shakes the theoretically-minded, knowledge-seeking trainee
and demands new tools brought to the field of study and of
conceptualization.

This rambling is leading me somewhere as I gather up the
various threads. And here is where I stand: A fellow at the
beginning of his training in child psychiatry faces an experience
which is unlike any experience he has had previously. To bring
this together with previous training by attempting to supply
continuities and consistencies and to translate or superimpose
theories may simply contribute to a paradox for the trainee such
as the one we intrdouced at the beginning--which class does he
belong in, if he does not believe that the classes themselves
are differentiated? Instead it seems better to focus on the
differences lest we encourage the trainees to make false
connections in their efforts to find continuities. Let me give
you a silly example. A little girl was brought by her parents
because after a fight with her mother she claimed to hear a
voice that told her to jump out the window. The therapist
pursued a line of questioning about the "voice," since if it is
the voice that is telling her to jump out the window, then the
only way to stop her from jumping out the window is to take care
of the voice. I think that if the issues are separated, the
treatment will proceed more effectively. The girl says she is
going to jump out the window, and she hears a voice. The more
pressing need is to prevent her from jumping out of windows.
If one uses a family approach, the parents, possibly the mother,
might be recruited for this responsibility, a struggle might
ensue in which the mother successfully prevents the child from
harming herself in this way, and the voice, having gone unnoticed

all this time may be forgotten.

        If we encourage our trainees to focus on the differences,
then we will encourage them to be receptive to novel situations,
open to extraordinary ideas, and we will have taught them how
to set a good paradox and how to escape from one.

FAMILY THERAPY AND CHILD PSYCHIATRY TRAINING: MAKING PEACE IN THE UNDECLARED WAR

Frederick M. Ehrlich, M.D.

Tufts University School of Medicine

Boston, Massachusettes

If one wants to know and understand a child, one needs to know and understand his family. This was obvious to Eric Erikson in 1950 when he described his custom of having dinner with the family of any child he considered treating--a custom so simple and sensible that it causes some embarrassment to acknowledge that it has been largely ignored. Not only is it unusual to have dinner with our patients' families, but it has been considered irrelevant and even harmful to meet with them at all.

Psychoanalysis has been interpreted, incorrectly I believe, as placing such primacy on the intrapsychic world that therapeutic modalities other than one-to-one contact were regarded as irrelevant. This misinterpretation fails to distinguish between psychoanalysis as a therapy which requires the patient and therapist to work together in isolation, and psychoanalysis as a theory and body of knowledge which can be applied more broadly and flexibly.

The advantages to child psychiatry of being able to see children and their families together have been stated clearly in articles (Malone, 1974; Zilbach, 1974; Ehrlich, 1973; and McDermott, 1974) and books (Skynner, 1976; Spiegel, 1971; Anthony, 1973). There is no need to repeat these arguments here, especially since ordinary common sense supports this view. However, an attempt to integrate a family approach into traditional psychoanalytic child psychiatric practice and training reveals profound difficulties. These difficulties can be divided into four overlapping areas: administration, teaching, technique, and theory. I shall consider some problems in each of these areas based on my experience.

Before beginning, we will need some definitions because many of the terms I use are used by different authors in different ways:

Psychoanalysis, psychoanalytic psychotherapy, and individual therapy--those forms of treatment of emotional disturbances based on an understanding of a dynamic unconscious as first described by Freud.

Psychoanalytic theory--the understanding of the body of knowledge of emotional development and function begun by Freud and including ego psychology and object relations theory. Although this theory considers man as a biological being and relates him to his environment, its primary focus is intrapsychic.

Family therapy--those forms of treatment of emotional disturbances that take the development and function of the entire family as their central focus, whether working with the family conjointly or with one or more members individually. The focus tends to be on current patterns of interaction.

Family theory--the body of knowledge of family emotional development and function. Work in this area relies heavily on systems, transactional, and communication theories (Skynner, 1976; Spiegel, 1971). There is nothing in family theory that is intrinsically incompatible with psychoanalytic theory.

Family interview or conjoint family interview--an interview in which three or more members of a family are seen in the same place at the same time.

Flexible family therapy--a form of treatment in which the focus may shift from the intrapsychic to the interactional and back again as required. The therapist or therapists may see the whole family or different members individually or in combinations.

I shall begin my discussion with problems of administration and teaching and then proceed to the underlying problems of practice and theory.

ADMINISTRATION

Although administrative issues are often considered mechanical and not worthy of serious thought, Ekstein and Wallerstein (1972) show that the setting of a training program, including the relationship between teachers and administrators and the structure of a clinic can have a vital effect on the work done (also see Stanton and Schwartz, 1954).

Administration has an appropriate concern about record-keeping. Traditionally, the child was the designated patient and all family material was kept in his/her record. In family therapy, since there may be no designated patient except the family, a separate chart is needed for each family member. These charts will be less complete than those of a child having a traditional evaluation, raising questions of responsibility and thoroughness. Unless these issues are worked through by the entire staff, the trainees are likely to get caught in the middle of a staff squabble.

Central to any clinical service is the process by which patients enter the service and disposition decisions are made. If a child is first evaluated individually and then the question of family treatment arises, one has already created a heavy bias toward individual therapy. If family therapy is to be integrated into clinical services, issues of the family must be considered from the very start and throughout the evaluation and treatment process. Unless the whole family is seen at the onset, there are many forces which press in favor of individual treatment. Among these forces are the greater familiarity and ease of arranging and keeping track of individual appointments, the inertia of the system, including clerical, administrative, and teaching staff, and the great anxiety most trainees feel when faced with family interviews.

I believe that issues of procedure have been among the most intransigent in our own clinic. Recently, a family with three children was referred to our Child Guidance Clinic by the Adult Inpatient Service where the father had been hospitalized. Concerns had been raised about all three children. The father's therapist favored an evaluation of the whole family together. The diagnostic supervisor, a staff member with a strong family orientation, accepted the trainee's preference to evaluate each child separately before having a family interview. The family interview, when it subsequently took place, led to a recommendation for time-limited conjoint family therapy. When questioned about her management of this case, the supervisor said that the trainees had been so apprehensive about seeing a family conjointly as the initial step that it had not been worth her effort to deal with it. The security of proceeding in the routine way interfered in this instance with a free use of clinical judgment.

Beal (1976) writes "The introduction of family therapy training into psychiatric centers organized along traditional lines...often creates disequilibrium and dysfunction." Jay Haley has been quoted as saying that it cannot be done without one or the other discipline being destroyed. I believe there is increasing evidence that Haley can be wrong, but only if administration is steadily supportive and open.

TEACHING

A mathematician once said that while a new concept may be agonizingly difficult for the teacher to integrate into his mathematical thinking, the same concept may be simple for students to whom it seems natural. Two competent senior psychiatrists in a mid-year discussion in a Family Therapy Seminar in which they had observed interviews with families agreed that they would not be brash enough to undertake conjoint family interviews. The two most junior members of the seminar, both social workers, later revealed that they were involved in a training program at a family institute and that each of them had several families in treatment.

This seminar was being offered at a Veterans Administration Outpatient Clinic with the hope that the staff could intervene directly with the children of the patients whom they had in treatment. The senior psychiatrists had joined the seminar because they were concerned about these children. By the end of the seminar year, we had arrived at the following conclusion: it would not be brash but wrong for them to undertake conjoint family interviews particularly where children were involved. They took their work seriously and were not going to undertake work for which they did not feel competent. They concluded that the seminar was useful in increasing their understanding of family dynamics and that it influenced their awareness of the children of their patients. It also became clear in case discussions that although these clinicians did not work directly with the children that they often made important interventions in the lives of these children through the work with their individual patients.

Let me compare this V.A. experience to the Child Guidance Clinic at Tufts-New England Medical Center. Here, for twelve years, trainees have been exposed to family theory and expected to conduct family interviews in addition to the individual therapy which is the central core of their training. In the program's first few years, trainees were apprehensive that they were caught in a power struggle between those teachers who did and those who did not "believe" in family interviews. There has gradually come to be a noncontroversial acceptance of family interviews as a means for understanding families, but considerably less agreement about this as a treatment modality. Some of this doubt is expressed openly; more of it appears indirectly in some of the administrative issues discussed earlier.

To assess the impact of this training, I wrote to the trainees who had graduated from our program over a period of five years. Seven of the ten replied. All but two use family interviews in their current work. These two are completing their adult psychiatry residencies, having taken their child psychiatry first, and say that they now have no opportunity to see families. Several, including those not currently seeing families, say that the family work in their training has influenced their understanding of individual patients.

One particularly thoughtful letter from a trainee, who now has significant teaching responsibility, outlines his exposure to family treatment in his training. As an adult resident, his thinking and interests were stimulated by a supervisor with whom he made home visits. He was then turned away from this interest by a respected teacher, an analyst, who described the desire to do family treatment as neurotically based. In the first year of his child psychiatry training at another center, his involvement with the families of child patients was mainly to get a history, after which the parents were seen by a social worker.

In his second year of child training at Tufts, he did not take the Family Therapy Seminar; his own family training was in supervision with me where he carried a "family case." He recalls being impressed when he discussed the case of a child brought to the emergency room by her whole family after attempting suicide, and I asked if he had used the opportunity to talk to the family. He realized that this had not occurred to him. He then describes how, stimulated by this rather small exposure to family therapy in his training, he has pursued this interest in his own thinking and clinical work. Finally, he states: "I see your influence in my training as important because I always viewed you as solidly skilled in individual work as well. In that sense, doing family work was not seen as an avoidance of the one-to-one contact, but rather, as a respected and valued alternative.... If I had had no teacher with an interest in and acceptance of family therapy, I very likely never would have pursued work that I think is a natural inclination for me."

I quote at such length not because this experience is atypical, but because I believe it is typical. A trainee need not be taught all areas of child psychaitry in equal depth, an impossible task, but he does need both exposure and an honest sense of inquiry and searching. While it has not been possible to integrate family work as solidly in our training program as some of us would like, it has had enough impact on the trainees that most of them have continued to pursue it on their own. Some of the trainees who have continued on as teachers are now deepening this work in their own teaching, and if it continues to make sense to more staff and trainees, the work and training in this area will grow in quality and extent.

TECHNIQUE

The task of learning psychoanalytic psychotherapy with child-

ren is surely one of the strangest in the world. To be open and
accessible to all details of feeling, both conscious and unconscious, without being intrusive, to remain aware of reality and
keeping things safe and under control without being controlling,
to keep still when it would be more natural to react and then to
say things which all our upbringing teaches us to keep silent
about--this is certainly enough to ask of our trainees. How can
we then ask them to undertake simultaneously family therapy
which requires contrary skills: to act and control, to intrude
and interfere, to make rules and correct errors, to focus on the
present and what is happening rather than on the past and what
has happened?

        Little wonder then that our first attempts at family therapy
in the Child Guidance Clinic created some turmoil. Family interviewing was seen by some as a peculiar and possibly dangerous
procedure; it was seen by others, myself included, as exciting
and experimental; still others saw it as exciting and wonderful,
but exotic, and possible only for a talented and free-wheeling
few, themselves not included.

        The situation now is changed. An integration of family
interviewing has occurred. This would not have been possible if
the differences in technique described earlier were accurate,
rather than exaggerations--the extreme positions of contending
groups. At present those who are most invested in a full
utilization of a family approach--particularly in a clinic with
rapid turnover of families with complicated socio-economic and
emotional problems--still complain that there is great resistance
and major administrative barriers to seeing families. On the
other hand, conjoint interviews are accepted as an ordinary
reasonable procedure.

        The trainees and younger staff may feel unskilled or anxious
in regard to family treatment, but they accept it as a sensible
procedure. Among older staff members, there are some who are
actively involved in family treatment and others who rarely or
never use this technique. This latter group is sometimes blamed
for undermining a vigorous family program by always focusing on
the individual dynamics in supervision and thereby putting the
trainee, who wants to do family work, in a bind.

        This is an unreasonable complaint. An experienced teacher
with great skill in work with individuals is going to teach what
he does most effectively and knows best. This becomes destructive
only if clinical approaches become a mask for political alignments
or if adherents are so rigid or shallow that they can consider
no alternative to their own work.

        Not so many years ago, child psychiatry training was unified

by an overwhelming emphasis on internal dynamics, and the approach
to theory and practice and teaching could be reasonably homo-
geneous. Today, a trainee must accept the stress of contending
points of view and priorities within his own program. This can
be fragmenting; on the other hand, it can also represent the
search for Truth that Milton describes in his <u>Areopagitica</u>. Truth
is compared to the body of Osiris dismembered and buried all over
Egypt to be searched out and reassembled by Isis, his sister,
before the god can be brought back to life. Each resident must
discover his own pieces of truth and attempt to assemble them
into his own coherent whole--the process of developing a therapeutic personality which Elvin Semrad (1969) said takes ten years
for a psychiatrist.

      The danger of turning out superficial, inadequately trained
individual therapists has always been great, and is increased now
by the growing demands on the curriculum. I do not agree, however,
with those who see family therapy as the enemy of individual
therapy, who see it as a <u>necessarily</u> manipulative approach to
people in which the power of transference relationship is misused
to impose the therapist's goals on the patient. I believe this
view confuses psychoanalysis with other forms of treatment. No
distinction is made between the impact of a therapist's words and
actions within an individual treatment session in which a
regressive transference is active, and the impact of words and
actions by a therapist in another setting or relationship. We
must not underestimate our patient's ability as well as our own to
assess reality. The power of the treatment relationship does not
depend on some mysterious, surgically clean field, but rather on
the individual impact at the level of relationship active between
patient and therapist during the therapy session.

      Our trainees can deepen their individual work if supervised
by teachers who understand and respect that work while simultaneously learning to deal with patients in the active here-and-now
technique of family intervention where that is appropriate.

      I now come to my central assertion: to effectively integrate
family therapy into child psychiatry training, at least some of the
teachers must do both individual and family treatment themselves
and teach and supervise both. The reason for this is not simply
one of mechanics or convenience, but is the deepest of all; only
someone who is integrating both theories and techniques in his
own work can teach in an integrated way. We ask a great deal of
our students, but we must not ask them to do our work for us. It
is part of our work to assess what is valuable in our field and
to present it in a coherent fashion. This does not mean that
we all have to agree, but that the core of any training program
must have sufficient integration so the trainee does not feel
he has to choose between incompatible views and hostile camps.

THEORY

Tanguay (1977) notes, "Say what you will about American child psychiatry, its heart has always been in the right place." But if we are to distinguish ourselves from the multitude of other good-hearted and therapeutically zealous, and justify our position in the medical and scientific community, we must remain open to all relevant information from whatever source and endeavor to reconcile discrepancies in our theories. We have an equal obligation to be pragmatic and do what works, and at the same time try to understand how it works and why it works. Since of all fields of medicine, ours is the most difficult in which to prove the efficacy of our methods, we have a particular obligation not to neglect our theory.

One problem that I see with the current field of family therapy is that we lose sight of this obligation. To return to Milton's (1967) analogy for the search for truth, I see Murray Bowen (1972) arriving with Osiris' left leg, the double bind group (Bateson, 1956) have his right leg, and Minuchin (1974) has dug up his heart and his liver. Each asserts with sincere conviction that he has found the Truth and that it works, but no one seems interested in fitting all the parts together and considering what is missing from the whole Osiris.

As child psychiatrists, we may have to remind our colleagues that there are not only biological, intrapsychic and environmental or interactional realities about which we know a great deal, but there also are developmental realities. The child at one age is very different from the child at another. Family therapy in some hands has treated all members as if they were adults and equals.

It is my impression that the most serious attempts to integrate psychoanalytic metapsychology and systems and trans-actional theory have been undertaken by adult psychiatrists—for instance the series of papers on projective identification by Berkowitz, Shapiro, Zimmer, and Shapiro (1974). Although the family is so obviously a central concern of child psychiatry, family theory has remained largely the province of people without primary knowledge of or immediate commitment to children.

What are some of the theoretical differences between a psychodynamic and a family system approach? Psychoanalysis says change comes through understanding; systems theory says understanding comes through change. Psychoanalysis says that if we correct the distortions of the past, we are free to deal accurately with present reality; systems theory says that if we correct present actions, the distortions of the past will be corrected.

Psychoanalysis says the ultimate reality is man alone; systems
theory says ultimate reality is man in interaction with his
environment. The apparent incompatability of these theories
disappears if we recognize that they need not be presented as
an either-or choice. One can consider that both this and that are
correct, but under different circumstances. In psychoanalysis,
we deliberately suspend interest in and contact with the outside
world in order to promote a regressive transference and agree
temporarily to suspend interest in any reality but the intrapsychic. This does not, or certainly should not, imply disdain
for, or a disbelief in the "real world." In conjoint family
therapy, when we focus on who is doing what to whom and the
confusion in the rules, we deliberately suspend interest in the
intrapsychic and act as if what people do or say is all that
matters. This need not, although it often does, imply a disdain
for or disbelief in intrapsychic reality.

There has been a remarkable parallel growth in many child
psychiatry training centers of what is called, by some, flexible
family therapy, in which there is a shift back and forth from the
individual to the family, from the intrapsychic to the interactional (Ehrlich, 1973; Malone, 1974; Skynner, 1976). This
growth has occurred, I believe, because it has made good sense
simultaneously to many teachers and practitioners, spurred in
part by students who keep asking questions. A period of "either-or"
is inevitable when the new challenges the old. If both prove
valuable, one can move into the less dramatic but more fruitful
stage of "both-and" which is where I believe we are now in regard
to family individual therapy and theory.

So we rediscover old truths--man is both alone and responsible
for himself, and a part of his emotional and physical environment.
Minuchin uses Milton's Paradise Lost as an example of the
presentation of Man as Hero. He quotes Satan recently thrown out
of Heaven:

>   The mind is its own place and in itself
>   Can make a Heaven of Hell, a Hell of Heaven

He dismisses this view of man as outmoded in our era of modern
physics and systems theory, an anachronism like romanticism or
psychoanalysis. What Minuchin forgets is that Milton did not ask
us to choose. Milton also presents this same Satan as quite
alterable by circumstances and part of the interactional field
in which he finds himself. Satan, the evil one, has arrived at
the Garden of Eden and entered the body of the serpent. He is
contemplating Eve, overawed by her beauty and innocent grace:

That space the evil one abstracted stood
From his own evil, and for the time remained
Stupidly good, of enmity disavowed
of guile, of hate, of envy, of revenge

CONCLUSION

If family theory and therapy, and psychoanalytic theory and
therapy are both true and useful, and I believe insofar as we are
able to understand the true and determine the useful that they
are, then we have a responsibility to include both in our practice
and teaching. I believe child psychiatry has a particular
opportunity to correct excesses and distortions and thereby to
bring a fuller understanding of both. There has been a remarkable
independent but parallel development in many training centers of
a similar form of family therapy which requires the ability to
work with and understand individuals and groups and the interactions between them. If we prove correct, our trainees, who are
exposed to improved depths and integration of these concepts early
in their training, will soon find many of our struggles to clarify
and integrate quite clumsy, because what has been new and
difficult for us, will be natural and easy for them.

REFERENCES

Anthony, E. J. and Koupernik, C. The Child in His Family. New
    York:Wiley, 1973.
Bateson, G., Jackson, D., Haley, J. and Weakland, J. Towards
    a theory of schizophrenia. Behavioral Science, 1, 251, 1956.
Beal, E. H. Current trends in the training of family therapists.
    American Journal of Psychiatry, 1976, 133:137-141.
Berkowitz, D., Shapiro, R., Zimmer, J. and Shapiro, E. Family
    contributions to narcissistic disturbances in adolescents.
    International Journal of Psychoanalysis, 1974, 1:353-362.
Bowen, M. Towards the differentiation of a self in one's own
    family. In: J. L. Framo, (Ed.) Family Interaction, New York:
    Springer, 1972.
Ehrlich, F. M. Family therapy and training in child psychiatry.
    Journal of American Academy of Child Psychiatry, 1973, 12:
    461-472.
Ekstein, R. and Wallerstein, R. The Teaching and Learning of
    Psychotherapy. New York:International Universities Press,
    1972.
Erikson, E. Childhood and Society. New York: Norton, 1963,
    pp. 53-54.
Malone, C. Observations on the role of family therapy in child
    psychiatry training. Journal of American Academy of Child
    Psychiatry, 1974, 13:437-458.

McDermott, J. and Char, W. The undeclared war between child and family therapy. Journal of American Academy of Child Psychiatry, 1974, 13:422-436.

Milton, J. Paradise Lost. 1667

Minuchin, S. Families and Family Therapy. Cambridge, Mass.: Harvard University Press, 1974, p.4.

Semrad, E. Teaching Psychotherapy of Psychotic Patients. David Buskirk, Ed.New York: Grune and Stratton, 1969.

Skynner, A. C. R. Systems of Family and Marital Psychotherapy. New York: Brunner/Mazel, 1976.

Spiegel, J. Transactions the Interplay between Individual, Family and Society. New York:Science House, 1971.

Stanton, A. and Schwartz, M. The Mental Hospital. New York:Basic Books, 1954.

Tanguay, P. Book review. Journal of Academy of Child Psychiatry, 1977, 16:540.

Zilbach, J. The family in family therapy. Journal of American Academy of Child Psychiatry, 1974, 13:459-467.

THE DYNAMICS OF THE WAR: DISCUSSION OF DR. EHRLICH'S PAPER

Fred Gottlieb, M.D.

University of California Los Angeles

Los Angeles, California

It is difficult for me to be critical of a person who cites John Milton and Elvin Semrad nicely in the same paragraph, and a person whose first name is also Fred! But I am critical of his presentation. As I understand it, Dr. Ehrlich confers both absolute and pragmatic truth value on both family system and psychoanalytic theory and therapy; he also pleads for "integration" --perhaps in deference to Dr. Brown's comments yesterday; we should now call this "Brownian synthesis!" As someone who struggled with the problem in physics of treating light sometimes as a wave form and sometimes as discrete particles, I can go along with an open and flexible theoretical view of the world. But heuristically we face serious problems which Dr. Ehrlich presents and then seems to sidestep. Early in his paper, he makes analytic theory schizophrenic: on the one hand he requires "patient and therapist to work together in isolation" and out of context, and on the other hand he says that "as a body of knowledge it can be applied more broadly and flexibly." Out in the West, we have a saying that goes, "You better put your money where your mouth is." Yesterday, Lee Combrinck-Graham said it differently: "Action speaks louder than words." Effective practice ought to reflect theory, or else we need to change the theory to better fit the data derived from revised practice.

As a respectful reader of Maxwell Gittleson, I know that analytic theoreticians have long dissected ants from the ant-hill, striving to maintain theory pristine and, concurrently, justifying modified or bastardized practice. I suggest the word "bastardized" here is a compliment rather than an epithet, because practice is and should be rooted <u>both</u> in theory <u>and</u> in the reality of having to be helpful to our patients. I think the latter is the more

crucial truth value test in our professional art. To paraphrase
Sinclair Lewis, truth is not a colored bird to be chased as it
hops or flies about. Truth or reality itself seems increasingly
suspect, appearing not as fixed but as variable, changing as a
function of perspective and context and time. When I wrote the
above, perhaps I felt out of patience with what I thought I might
have mistaken for an individual treatment and/or psychoanalytic
apologia. Having heard Dr. Ehrlich's discussion of Dr. Combrinck-
Graham's paper yesterday, I now realize that I did not misunderstand
him.

     I was appreciative of Dr. Ehrlich's candor with respect to
his own clinic and personnel's problems in achieving and maintaining a family perspective. I do not think he is correct when
he calls these intransigent difficulties "issues of procedure";
and as he confirmed later in his paper such issues are mere
reflections of his own institutional or system-specific orientation.
I also was pleased with Dr. Ehrlich's analogy concerning mathematical concepts and how sometimes it's simpler for the generation
which follows than it was for the pioneer creators and teachers.
Similarly, it is clear to me that effective family therapists and
teachers whom I know often are excellent when seeing an
individual, that is, in doing and teaching individual work. If
the reverse were true, we might not need this symposium! But alas,
few individual therapists are expert in family work. The reason
is not merely training, I think, but has to do with core orientation. The family therapist working with an individual always
keeps the interpersonal context in mind, rather than focusing
exclusively or predominantly on intrapsychic issues. That
distinctive orientation is hard to gainsay, although I think that
Dr. Ehrlich nobly tried to do so.

     Dr. Ehrlich's prose about Milton, Satan, Eve, and the Garden
of Eden, deserves a response. I chose a slightly different
literature, but maintained the setting. Early in the 1900's,
there was a private gathering of about 100 of the most influential
persons in a large American city. Lincoln Steffens was there,
talking with them. In his autobiography he describes his thesis
for the evening, really a synopsis of his life-long view. He
had begun in his early muckraking thinking that bad men,
especially bad politicians, caused bad government; the politicians,
whom he found were really rather decent individually, in turn
blamed the business men to pressured or bribed them. Upon inquiry,
the business men, just like the politicians, were not really bad
people. It turned out that regardless of character, education,
or station, people in certain businesses were in the business of
the corruption of politics and the resistance to reform. Steffens
described to the group that it is not the persons themselves, but
it is the way society is organized. He says "we have an

organization of society in which the...ablest most resourceful
leaders...are...against society('s) laws...."

   The first question from that company and the last was "Who
started the evil?" A kindly bishop asks at the end, "Who
founded the system...in the beginning?"   Steffens' answer, long
before we used such words as linear versus circular causality,
or spoke of open system thinking, comes to the heart of the issue
for all of us: He responds "Well, Bishop, you want to fix the
fault at the very start of things. Most people say it was Adam.
But Adam...said that it was Eve...and Eve said no, no, it wasn't
she; it was the serpent. And that's where you clergy have stuck
ever since. You blame that serpent, Satan. Now I come and I am
trying to show you that it was, it is, the apple."

   Like all metaphors, this one too may suffer in application
to our own situation. But clearly, we in psychiatry face a
system problem. And it is not merely the presence of or the
strength of individual ego psychologists and/or child analysts or
behavior modifiers who encumber our proclamations of truth, at
least as we see "truth." Looking just one level beyond, we are
all involved in a much more complex system called "medical
education"; in that system we are all, to varying degrees, the
corrupted and the corrupters. With Dr. Ehrlich's help in bringing
up Satan and the Garden of Eden, and here in New York (the
"Big Apple") I hope you will forgive me for repeating Steffens'
metaphor of the apple, of the system itself being the issue.
Anyway, I hope that apple will provide some food for your thought.

THE TENSION THAT RESULTS FROM AN INTEGRATED APPROACH: GENERAL

DISCUSSION

<u>AUDIENCE MEMBER</u>

Is there a need for evil in order to define ourselves? Is
there a need to perceive individual therapy as an evil in order
to define family therapy? Is there a need to perceive family
therapy as an evil in order to define individual therapy? Is
it going to be the individual therapist versus the family therapist?
Are we going to spend all of our time today and down through the
corridors of time debating this, fighting with each other? Can
we really put it together in some way that is meaningful and
useful, defining what we do, not on the basis of the split, but
just on what we do? And, can we in some way encompass it all in
a unity which comes back to the idea of one approach?

<u>DR. MALONE</u>

To some extent, it is a matter that some people focus on
differences and some people focus on similarities. There are the
educators who look for ways of attempting to integrate diverse
viewpoints. There are those who can learn most, or perhaps contribute most, by looking at differences. As far as the papers
presented here are concerned, a lot of the very real and important
issues to be discussed have not really been addressed that clearly
or directly, and that is unfortunate.

There are some points of integration and there are obviously
some points of difference, and neither has been explored particularly in this whole process. This is not exactly an accident,
because there are very tough issues that still remain to be
explored. They certainly remain to be explored in terms of
research. In some ways, it is an inevitable thing in terms of the
current state of the art. The process of really getting at some
of these issues is going to take a lot of very hard work. As many
people have said, when you try to maintain an integrated field,
there are considerable tensions which all of us experience. I
think that is part of the reason why we sometimes choose to move

conceptually to a viewpoint which is most comfortable for us,
whatever that happens to be.

DR. EHRLICH

I very much appreciate Dr. Gottlieb's comments because they
sharpened something for me. He said almost in passing, something
very important. In his experience, the best family therapists are
also good individual therapists, but that the best individual
therapists are generally not good family therapists. Clearly,
I believe implied in this statement is that he sees family therapy
as more effective in general.

If that is true, and I am willing to concede that it may
be true, the most effective therapy going on is by family
therapists. I say to Dr. Gottlieb and to all of us, prove it.
And that is where we are. Maybe this is one of Dr. Malone's issues
of importance. We need, if it is possible, outcome studies. I
say if it is possible, because I am not at all convinced that it
is. We may be talking about measuring intrinsically different
things. But I do think at least we need to ask. Can there be
good outcome studies? What do we want to measure? And either
agree that we can measure it and go about the business of saying
that those who have had strict family training as their primary
orientation do better work at it, or not? After all, I have seen
enough failures in my own work and humble enough about our
capacity to change that if anyone can show that a particular
approach is going to really be more effective in altering the
misery of the lives of children and making them grow better, I am
all for it.

The point I will not yield on at all is that the internal
world, as revealed and known only to some extent, in individual
self-contemplation or in the psychoanalytic situation, is a real,
important, enduring part of human beings and human experience. It
may be irrelevant to therapy. I do not think so, but it may turn
out 50 years from now, people will say that is a fascinating way
to study people, but it does not alter them. Again, I do not
think so, but is is possible. I will not yield that it is a
part of us. It is data that can be obtained no other way, and it
is a terribly important aspect of what makes us human and we need
to know about its development in children and understand it whether
we use it directly in our treatment or not.

IDENTITY, TRAINING AND GROWTH: FAMILY THERAPY AND TRAINING CHILD

PSYCHIATRISTS

Fred Gottlieb, M.D.

University of California Los Angeles

Los Angeles, California

I. THE STUDENTS

The youngest enter the fellowship at age 27 or 28. Many are
30, beginning the fourth decade of their lives, still in training
and still seeking their niche of professional identity. Some
come to child psychiatry because their past experiences with
children had been particularly rewarding. They may have forged
important bonds with younger siblings or cousins, worked re-
wardingly in summer children's camps, or functioned well with
pediatric patients; perhaps some successfully tutored disadvantaged
youngsters, or empathically counseled kids in trouble. Others
come with less experience and consequently with even more ideal-
istic fervor: "Children are the future! Give me the child and
I'll give you the adult! As the twig is bent, so the tree
grows!" Some Child Fellows are wary of adults, feel more secure
with children. A few seek to re-parent themselves.

For still others, work in child psychiatry stems from psychoanalytic interests. Symptomatic dis-ease is seen as a result of
conflict between the psychic components. Such conflicts should
be more transparent and, therefore, more readily remediable before
they become concealed in the confusing overgrowth of subsequent
developmental stages and additional complicated life experiences.
Rather than doing long retrospective analyses with careful unfolding
of historical layers and structures, they see the child in status
nascendi, readily recruited for rapid return to a healthier
developmental pathway.

A few older trainees have entered psychiatry after working
in other medical areas. Often these are people who began medicine

with great humanistic strivings, but took a wrong turn somewhere between the dialysis machine and the MA-2 Respirator or the stack of Schwan-Ganz catheters. In their rush to rescue the patient, sometimes they lost sight of him. They may turn to psychiatry in order to recoup, to work with the whole patient, not just a disease syndrome. In adult psychiatry, they find an old linear system catechism often awaits them. Perhaps the child program seems different, more humanistic, more hopeful, less overtly voyeuristic or somehow less tawdry.

In any event, this heterogeneous group arrives in child fellowship programs at a national rate of 250 per year, with some disillusioned about medicine, or about adult psychiatry, or about parents; others eager with many illusions about children, developmental psychology, child analysis, or their own potential potency. The incoming Child Fellow already is lengthily trained, at least seven years beyond college graduation, thrust once again into a student role just at a time when he or she finally is consolidating some sense of competent professionalism as a psychiatrist. Child psychiatry programs carefully protect the Fellows' emerging psychiatric identity. Training in child psychiatry is portrayed as a natural extension of the adult psychiatric work which the fellow has already experienced. The notion of a treatment team, previously present in more cursory form in adult work, now is emphasized and extended to include a variety of other professionals in education, psychology and social work. The titular team leader is a child psychiatrist or Child Fellow, knowledgeable or not. The trainee experiences a ritual induction into an organized power hierarchy which confers upon him both status and money perquisites and helps support the process of professional identity consolidation.

II. PROFESSIONAL IDENTITY

The psychoanalytic term identity has a complicated and precise meaning which refers to psychic organization as it develops in successive life phases, and which is partly unconscious. In this paper, as did Allen Wheelis (1958) a score of years ago in his book The Quest for Identity, I refer to identity in its ordinary meaning, that is, as a coherent sense of self: "I'm a man; I'm a psychiatrist; I'm a husband, a father; a fine therapist; a feeling person; a secular Jew; an American; a Californian." Identity clarity derives from stable values and from the dependable linkage of one's actions with one's values. Thus, identity clarity reflects a sense of wholeness or integrity. In a well-functioning family and society, individual identity both grows out of and also validates the belief that one's efforts in life make sense or are meaningful in context.

For many aerospace engineers and applied physicists who had
faith in the human benefits to be derived from advancing technology,
it has become more difficult to sustain their earlier and more
certain identity. A similar issue exists for assembly line
workers who begin to discount their routinized work efforts as
meaningless, or for theologians who become less certain in their
faith, or for psychiatrists if we question some of our own,
previously basic, tenets. Thus, as Western society discards the
absolute primary of linear thinking, the fixed reference points
of past certainties are lost. Cause and effect become intertwined. Educator and student, designated therapist and other
therapy participants, become joined in a more complex system.
Such a conceptual shift is particularly relevant for a trainee
in child psychiatry exposed to a family system point of view.

Let us consider the situation of the Child Fellow. As
Sharaf and Levinson (1964) pointed out 15 years ago, the dynamic
psychiatrist in training tries to master a complex field while
concurrently carrying major life responsibility for a number of
patients. Such a situation may generate considerable anxiety
about therapeutic potency and stimulate some of the polar
behaviors we often see in the trainee. There are those who are
somewhat panicky, shy away from patient contact, seem reluctant
to assume responsibility, cannot readily arrange to schedule
patients for a live supervision session or an interview; instead,
they become busier reading articles or books, doing charts,
attending seminars and staff meetings, or otherwise participating
in myriad available activities not directly clinical. Other
residents outwardly manifest great confidence and plunge quickly
into terribly complicated treatment situations with naive earnest-
ness. They seek out the supervisor for additional time, may ask
for special cases, actively manifest much excitement about the
new experience. Although they believe they are doing things in
a new way, just as they had been instructed, these are sometimes
the very trainees who find it most difficult actually to shift to
alternative intervention patterns.

Most trainees fall between those extremes. Whichever are
their personally preferred styles of adjusting to the new and
stressful learning situation, all are motivated by more-or-less
mature aspirations for competence and mastery. Faced with
relative inexperience with children, the trainee is sometimes
very self-critical. First accurately and then often with
exaggeration, he perceives several persons in the training program
who stand out as particularly knowledgeable or clinically skillful.
Professional expertise and potential membership in the guild of
child psychiatrists becomes available through responsible hard
work and concurrently through rational use of role models as
sources of competence, mentors to whom one can apprentice. As

teachers, we are aware that students often also harbor irrational
ideas about the mentor with whom the trainee identifies, a mentor
who then is imbued with unique and remarkable potency.

Processes of imitation and identification are not limited
to those we view as formal students, but also occur naturally with
our children, our friends, our patients and other colleagues.
Seventeen years ago when I did individual work with psychotic
patients on a closed ward, I smoked a pipe; I noticed a number
of my patients became pipe-smokers for a time during treatment.
A few months ago, my wife picked me up at the airport after a
weekend conference where I had spent some time with Sal Minuchin.
We were talking as we threaded our way home through heavy traffic,
when she chuckled: "You're talking just like Sal." She was
referring to an unmistakably identical cadence and lilt in my
speech after being with the charismatic Minuchin. Such temporary
imitations and partial identifications occur in more important
ways than merely smoking a pipe or polyglot aftermath of accent,
intonation, body posture, or word choice. Such imitations are
significant as forerunners of and accompaniments to those important
changes we work toward as teachers. We are interested in our
students' affective and behavioral and cognitive integration:
We are interested in their professional identity. Imitation is
not only the sincerest form of flattery, but also provides a
highly visible marker for those necessary incorporative processes
on route to genuine identification and professional identity
consolidation.

As a family therapy supervisor, I make sure that students
can observe my own work with families, as well as when I
directly intervene in the treatment of families assigned to them.
Early in my trainees' experience in videotape supervision,
occasionally one of them presents a segment of his tape work with
a comment on the order of: "Now what's coming is a Gottlieb
maneuver." A few years ago when that happened, I felt annoyed.
My own student identity had persisted. I felt that the credit
given was wrong, that they should have recognized it was really
a "Minuchin maneuver!" Later, in clarifying my own identity as
a teacher, and of method rather than style, I became perplexed
that they didn't see that the particular maneuver was grounded in
a body of theory, that it was a "structural family therapy
maneuver!" Nowadays I am less concerned, but still remain alert
to the developmental aspects of such remarks. I know that, at
least for some Child Fellows, it is only a matter of time and
experience: Soon they will present tape segments without using
the language of imitation and partial identification with a
mentor, nor cognitive terms merely reflecting incorporation of a
theoretical body of knowledge. Instead, they will say to me and
to their peers in supervision, "Let me tell you how I thought
about the problem and worked it out; and let me show you what I

did about it in this session." They will have begun to come to
terms with their own identity as child psychiatrists who work
with families. Our job as teachers is to help bring about such
growth.

III. THE TRAINING CONTEXT

     Child psychiatry training occurs predominantly in the "aca-
demic centers" of American psychiatry, i.e., university-affiliated
programs, usually in departments headed by adult psychiatrists.
Divisions of Child Psychiatry have grown slowly in such programs,
often have been challenged to demonstrate the unique worth of
child psychiatry, have had to scramble for departmental and
governmental funds and sometimes to fight for survival itself in
the internecine struggles of academia.

     Family therapy is a relative newcomer on the professional
mental health scene. Once considered a possible meeting ground
for child and adult psychatrists, it still may fulfill that
function, but not in the rather simplistic way traditional
child psychiatrists initially imagined. As McDermott (1974)
noted, for a long time textbooks in child psychiatry did not even
list family therapy as a treatment modality: child journals
printed only a few limited and cautiously descriptive articles
on interviewing, not therapy, or reviewed books in the family
field. The traditional view (an ancillary worker keeps the
parents out of the way to lessen "reinfection" by them and to
prevent disruptions while the psychiatrist actually treats the
child) continued in action even while sensible child psychiatrists
were urging, on good theoretical grounds, that we should be paying
a lot of attention to the family. But "paying attention" remained
quite apart from viewing the family as a functional unit for
evaluation and intervention. McDermott said Child Psychiatry once
was treated as a step-child housed in adult psychiatric training
programs. I would extend the metaphor: family therapy, when allowed
in the house at all, clearly was an offensive or disreputable
relative, tolerated because of remote but undeniable consanguinity.

     With adult psychiatry's grudging recognition of the need for
and import of specialized child psychiatric skills and developmental knowledge, child psychiatry has obtained space in which to
mature. And when child psychiatrists say that an _essential_ in
basic child psychiatry is expertise in interviewing, understanding,
and formulating issues and interventions from a family perspective,
there is evidence that maturation is occurring. McDermott's
"war" is past.

     In the spirit of Camp David, we have curricular peace treaties
and coexistence in many training programs. But I suggest that the

historical and continually pervasive influence of child analysis
on child psychiatry training may make genuine rapproachement
unlikely. When family work occupies a minimal few hours in the
curriculum, or when there are only a few experienced family
clinicians and teachers on a sizeable faculty, we raise our eye-
brows. When observation rooms for direct supervision are inadequate, or when videotape machinery and tapes are unavailable,
we grow restive.

The distinctive conceptual framework and application of
family diagnosis and intervention differentiates family therapy
increasingly from traditional adult and child psychiatry. Trainees
come to a Child Fellowship with certain skills, are pleased as
well as apprehensive about their entry into child psychiatry,
and begin the process of skill development and identity re-
crystalization which I described earlier. Their usual difficulties
are more complex when there is a major conceptual division of the
faculty. One example is the split between these child psychiatrists
who teach the trainee to approach problems from an individual
perspective and those who approach from a family systems perspective.

The split is immediately evident, manifest with the first
clinical assignment, the first evaluation interview: Is it
scheduled for an individual child, or separately for the identified
patient and one accompanying adult, or for the whole family? Is
the clinic's charge different for an hour's family session than
for another professional hour? Are there institutionaly approved
ways to chart family data? Do the personnel accept videotape
usage routinely and convey that to the incoming help-seekers?
These questions are trivial, except insofar as they reflect on
the institution's and training program's values, on the faculty's
approach and de facto identity.

In passing, let me suggest that it may become necessary to
achieve a critical mass, a "sufficient" number of family therapists
to have effective impact within a program. Now I'll present some
personal observations and experiences regarding teaching of family
therapy within the program in which I work. The overall training
context is centrally significant but obviously differs for every
institution. Perhaps some of the experiences I am going to
present may provide you some ideas which may be applicable for
implementation within the programs in your own institutions.

IV. PERSONAL OBSERVATIONS ON TEACHING FAMILY WORK

The Neuropsychiatric Institute at the University of California,
Los Angeles, (UCLA-NPI) offers a large general psychiatry residency

program, with rotations both at the base hospital and in two nearby
Veterans Administration Hospital settings. There are four children's wards at UCLA NPI itself, with bed space for approximately
80 children and adolescents. The child outpatient service
records some 14,000 patient visits per year. The Division of
Mental Retardation and Child Psychiatry has a large program
component in mental retardation, which provides additional funding
for training a substantial number of nonpsychiatric professionals,
e.g., social work students, graduate nurses, psychology interns,
other physicians, etc. Seven to ten Child Psychiatry Fellows
graduate from the training program each year. Before 1976, family
therapy training for the latter was available through participation
in a 1 1/2 hour weekly seminar for eight months of the first
Fellowship year. In addition to discussion of articles and
presentation of family therapy films, this seminar time also was
used to provide opportunity for case supervision for those trainees
(usually paired) who were treating "family cases." In the past
several years, a number of changes have occurred within the
teaching program. I shall comment upon some of the issues,
strategies, and continuing problems in gradually changing the
training so that it might become more significant in the total
teaching program and a more effective learning vehicle for the
Child Fellows.

A.   The Didactic Teaching Sequence

    General systems theory posits that an equivalent end state
results from the same operations within a system no matter what
the sequence of the operations. But the chemistry of human interaction is such that sequence, although perhaps not everything,
is quite a critical variable! For example, we can utilize the
identity fluidity of beginning Child Fellows in order to gain
access before the Fellows lock onto those traditional individual
strategies of intervention with children which increase resistances
to learning a family approach. In 1976 I started the Family
Therapy seminar after the Fellows had been in the program ten
weeks; they had already become experienced ("indoctrinated?") in
starting an evaluation by usually seeing one parent first, taking
a detailed chronological and developmental history very early and
relatively formally, then seeing the child individually for a
number of sessions etc. Now I begin the Family Seminar earlier
in the Fellowship. This simple shift seems very helpful. Were
the program generally more oriented to family evaluation and
intervention, such an artifice would be unnecessary.

    Initially, I presented didactic material spread over many
months, but the Fellows began to see families and have supervision during the very same week their seminar began. While
children may learn to swim by being dropped into the water, this

is not a pleasant experience for the teacher or the learner. In
response to the Fellows' urgings, now I give a preparatory series
of ten sessions (15-20 hours) during their first or second month
in training, which functions cognitively and affectively to gear
them up, to calm some of their anxieties about this "new" approach,
and even whet the appetites of some who become eager to try out
what they are learning. They are assigned patients and supervisory
time at the end of this preparatory set of seminars. The first
ten sessions of preparation and the first year's mandatory
supervision are both based upon structural family theory.

As part of the learning sequence, the Fellows have ten
additional sessions at six months into the program in order to
learn about a number of alternative family therapy models. The
final mandatory "academic" experience is for them to participate
in another ten sessions during the final three months of their
first year, during which they each select an area of family work
to study intensively and to report to their colleagues in the
seminar. In the near future, I am planning several elective
courses: One is a course looking at theories of change; another
is a short series of sessions on improvisation, led by an ex-actor,
now family therapist! Later these may become part of a formal
sequence within the second Fellowship Year.

B.   Training with Whom?

"Belonging" to an "externally" identifiable group is an
important aspect of "internal" identity formation. The group
provides validation for one's person, values and actions, helps
confirm a psychic core of identity. Child Fellows often come
into family work lacking the formal preparation and sophistication
of many other trainees. Sometimes they appear unaware of their
deficits in knowledge and the traditional medical hierarchy may
function to perpetuate a number of their prejudices born of
ignorance. One prejudice is that the psychiatrist is, ipso
facto, a better dynamic clinician than other mental health
professionals. Another prejudice is that traditional individual-
based psychodynamic theory is, ipso facto, both a necessary and
also sufficient explanation for those observable human problems
labelled "psychopathology." Part of my early training effort is
to disrupt both these prejudices and yet not too vigorously shake
the Fellow's emerging professional identity.

One strategy is to utilize an expanded social system to
place pressure on the Fellows to consider interpersonal rather than
traditional formulations. For example, in 1978's preparatory
seminars, I embedded seven first-year Child Fellows within a
larger group of trainees of varying status: 11 psychology interns,
three faculty physicians from the Family Practice residency

program, several postdoctoral students from psychology and
anthropology, and a number of experienced nurses and social
workers. Partly to maintain some necessary degree of specialness
for the Fellows, periodically I alluded positively to their
coherence as a training group and to their forthcoming unique
supervisory arrangements.

In general, the observations made by the anthropologist,
comments by the Family Practice faculty, and the questions raised
by the postgraduate psychologists were extremely valuable for the
entire seminar. The collegial setting and verbal sharing, and
the alternative perspectives posed by others expert in their fields,
helped organize the Fellows to think through issues, without
placing them in a situation which might somehow oblige them either
to defend individual treatment orthodoxy or to accept a family
systems bandwagon uncritically. For a while they sat back a bit.
As the month progressed, they become more activated in the sessions,
full participants who asked questions and freely commented. Of
added interest, they did not become engaged in polemics or other
resistances to approaching problems from a family systems perspective. The Fellows seemed to accept a role as a respected
subset of students amongst a more heterogeneous group. I think
the setting helped facilitate their learning.

C. Supervision

Group size, etc. The underlying notion in my program is
that change occurs experientially. Family members experience
alternative interpersonal ways of relating. Similarly, supervision in this model should develop experiential skills in the
therapist. Beyond increasing specific skills, frequently there
are important supervisory by-products. These include the Fellows'
developing a generally more positive view of humankind, a lessening
of pathology-hunting, and increasing comfort and ease with warmth
and other empathically experienced affects. At different times,
I have provided family supervision to trainees as individuals,
in pairs, and in groups of three and four. Issues may more
frequently arise in one particular supervisory format compared to
another. The traditional notion in individual dynamic supervision
is that the supervisory experience replicates the therapeutic
experience. Concepts of transference/counter-transference/resis-
tance, etc., then are applied to the supervisory situation. If
the model were used that supervision replicates therapy, one
would not see an individual, but would create a "trainee family"
group, ready to explore small-group dynamics and personal issues
as they come up in supervision. I believe there may be validity
to this approach, but don't think it is an efficient way to
develop the trainee's specific experiential skills. In such a
family group, as in a one-to-one arrangement, the supervisor also

more often feels the pull to try to be therapeutic with the trainee.

There are many reasons that family therapy supervisors
usually eschew regular supervision of just one trainee. And it
is not only because we are reluctant to cast supervisorial
brilliance before a single person rather than an admiring covey.
A single trainee just is not exposed to the spectrum of therapeutic styles and interactions he or she would see if colleagues
regularly presented work in supervision. That provides a greater
range of family problems, stimulating both for students and for
the supervisor! Performance pressure is less for any one trainee
when others are present to share their own difficulties. When a
"weaker" Fellow is in solo supervision, there may be a greater
tendency for the supervisor to intervene to protect the family
instead of allowing the resident time to work it out. And
occasionally the supervisor gets into a kind of cycle, where he
sees the Fellow's work through blinders, repetitively critical in
a way which is not useful. This may diffuse out more readily
when several other trainees are present, rather than just the
supervisor and one trainee, who have become choreographed into a
"more of the same" sequence.

There are also difficulties with a single trainee who is
very "good," often when the supervisor begins to enjoy fantasies
of a kind of protege relationship. The supervisor's espectations
may become unrealistic. The Fellow does something status-
appropriate but which is disappointing to the supervisor. It's
fine to walk on water until you make a misstep. The supervisor
may feel perturbation, or chagrin, but either way, the teaching
suffers. Sometimes, particularly when working alone with such a
"good" resident, the supervisor is tempted to overlook small
issues because of the halo-effect of the Fellow's other fine
work. Such problems continue and worsen without adequate
supervisory resolution.

I did one hour supervision sessions with each of five pairs
of Fellows during a six-month period last year. My conclusion:
Don't do it that way! One supervision hour is ample time for
one Fellow to present, but really isn't enough for two Fellows.
Essentially what happened is the pair alternated sessions for
presentation of tapes. Of both theoretical and practical concern
was the more frequent emergence of triangulation patterns in a
few of these groups. For a time with one pair, I found myself
in coalition with one of the trainees. I observed how we two
worked synchronously, and not just to be helpful to the other
trainee, but subtly putting him "in the back of the supervisory
bus." As you might guess, that trainee was himself well practiced
in preferring that position and he had played out his role in
our systemic replication. The potential dyadic rivalry of the
two Fellows may facilitate such discoveries. But for that trainee

to experience himself as respectably assertive should <u>not</u> require
that early in the supervision he take a secondary position to
that of his colleague.

Another pair supported each other's resistance patterns to
doing family work. One or another would come late, miswork the
tape machine, help families make appointment times when they
could not be taped, be unable to locate newly assigned families
for a week or two, etc. For a while I was clearly the odd-one-out
in this triangle.

Pair supervision often is <u>effective</u>, but the supervisor
must consider its relative inefficiency: the addition of a third
trainee provides a 50% increase in trainee exposure to family
experiences and to supervisory suggestions. With three trainees
in a 1 1/2 hour supervisory session, two present each week.
Sometimes they split the time evenly, sometimes one asks for
more time, in which case the other has priority the next week.
Naturally, the same problems I've described previously can occur
in groups of three trainees, but they seem less likely or less
marked. With a group of four trainees, two present material
each week, 45 minutes to one hour each, depending on the overall
session length. In the first part of the year I now schedule
two-hour supervision blocks, whether with three or four trainees,
both because we can always use the time and also because I can
do more live supervision then without having to schedule it for
another time. Sometimes just keeping track is hard with four
trainees in one supervisory session. I recommend reviewing the
supervisory notes beforehand, as one would review therapy notes
before a family session.

Early in the trainees' year I am reluctant to have visitors
present at supervision. Later in the year I feel freer to invite
visitors, and the Fellows appear to appreciate their presence.
The Fellows make efforts to explain and seem pleased to show their
work. I've had several long-stay foreign visitors, whom I
thought were most helpful. In one pair-supervision, a visiting
Italian's presence helped rearrange the structure as she joined
one member of a resistant dyad but kept distance from the other.
In another supervision, an Israeli psychologist participated for
many months. Sometimes I was heard better by the students when
I addressed my comments to them indirectly by talking to the
Israeli. And, of course, visiting colleagues sometimes can help
us to break out of stereotypic supervisory molds when they ask
questions or make observations from a perspective different from
the one to which we've become accustomed.

I've had Psychology Interns together with Child Fellows in
supervision and thought it worked reasonably well. Afterwards
the Fellows said they preferred keeping their own professional

group intact. I think they are probably correct, for reasons
suggested earlier in this paper. This year I am supervising a
postdoctoral psychologist with one group of three Child Fellows.
The postdoc also is doing camera work for many of the Child
Fellows, which I think has joined them more readily.

   Retrospective videotape and live supervision. Of all the
strange notions new Child Fellows are exposed to, live supervision seems to be the most affectively troubling. When I first
show them a tape of me being interrupted by a supervisor, they
seem to laugh with apprehension and delight, embarrassment and
pleasure. "You're kidding...you mean you'll interrupt us?" They
are surprised at the relief they experience when the supervisor
phones in, or better yet, comes into the room when they are
having too difficult a time. And they are astonished at the
ease with which the families accept this intrusion, and then
resume their discussion with the assigned therapist moments later.
The families' acceptance of a staff member calling or coming in
sets the tone which may help the therapist to accept it.

   For the trainees, live supervision has been one of the
most powerful tools in learning family therapy skills and in
appreciating experiential rather than verbal change. When an
experienced supervisor intervenes in a family session to activate
an alternative transactional pattern between family members, the
trainee sees and feels first-hand the power of the tools available
to him. Although the trainee has seen many videotapes of other
therapists and me, there is something very special when I go into
the room with the trainee and the family. "I never realized how
softly you spoke" is a comment I hear frequently from trainees
who may have viewed incisive segments on videotape but have not
fully realized these can occur only when there is a solid joining
of therapist and family, on ongoing respectful linkage. Rarely
a therapist will feel "You came in too soon. I was getting to
the same place." And occasionally, a Fellow who is foundering
aimlessly activates the supervisor to an extraordinary and heroic
intervention, afterwards only to say blandly, "Oh yes, you did
xyz, that was interesting...." A few weeks or months later the
supervisee may recall that time with appropriate intensity.

   Because of time constraints on the supervisor, only a limited
amount of live supervision is feasible. I try to do more of it
at the beginning of training, and over the year also give phone
directions in preference to going into the therapy room itself.
Retrospective videotape supervision seems adequate, as well as
offering certain advantages, e.g., to replay certain particularly
informative or uncertain segments. When staff or second-year
Fellows arrange for a live supervision session, they expect me

to come in, perhaps as an acknowledgement that the problem was
tough enough to arrange the session. Since we've recently
introduced a very large one-way mirror in the family taping room,
it is more obvious how two-dimensional the tape is, compared to
really being on the scene in the room itself. Our trainees do
usually videotape themselves. But despite careful instruction
at the onset of supervision, about half the trainees manage to
foul up one tape, often simply by not pressing the proper buttons
to begin a recording. For the few trainees who do not solve such
"mechanical" issues promptly, it has signaled a difficult supervisorial experience.

   Teaching staff colleagues. In the past several years, I
have introduced concepts of structural family therapy to 20 or 30
members of our staff and other professional colleagues in the
community. Many of these have incorporated this way of approaching
issues into their work; some of the social work staff in the UCLA
Medical Center and the NPI Gerontology ward and in the UCLA Family
Practice Center have utilized live supervision to develop their
skills experientially. Medical faculty members have been involved,
too, from the Family Practice, Adult Psychiatry, Geriatric
Psychiatry, and Human Sexual Dysfunction programs. Faculty from
the Division of Child Psychiatry have been invited, indicated
interest, but, with one exception, have always pleaded time
pressure to justify their decision not to attend. By arranging
such in-service training for our faculty on alternate weeks this
coming Spring to replace a regularly scheduled administrative
meeting, perhaps now we will achieve significant Child Psychiatry
Faculty exposure.

   I don't think we who are teachers of family therapy in child
psychiatry training programs need to feel paranoid about our own
colleagues' resistance to change, but it is real; it is understandable and it is justified. Family therapy is a natural
extension of child psychiatry's evolving appreciation of the
child's surroundings. We looked at the mother and the school or
other environment; a little later we included the father; and now
finally we try to view in a more comprehensive context. But in
addition to being evolutionary, family therapy also is perceived
correctly as revolutionary. In its perspective shift from
individual intrapsychic pathology to systemic interpersonal
functioning, in its emphasis on current experiential change rather
than insightful understanding, and in its focus on the therapist
as an active part of the process rather than a passive, neutral
observer/interpretor, family therapy disrupts some of the time-
honored foundations of the profession. When the teaching methodology involves regular use of one-way mirrors, videotape and
access into the therapy room by the supervisor, our colleagues
draw back a bit.

But in my opinion, it is this very area which is most
important for our symposium. It is only after we have had working
impact on our <u>faculty</u> colleagues, not via exhortative proselytizing
but by direct exposure and first-hand experience, that family
therapy concepts and skills then will be <u>genuinely</u> integrated
into the training of every child psychiatrist.

REFERENCES

Allen, J. D. Peer group supervision in family therapy. <u>Child
    Welfare</u>, 55, 183-189, 1976.
Beal, E. W. Current trends in the training of family therapists.
    <u>American Journal of Psychiatry</u>, 133, 2, 137-141, 1976
Bodin, A. M. Videotape applications in training family therapists.
    <u>Journal of Nervous and Mental Disease</u>, 148, 251-261, 1969
Brody, E. B. Models in psychiatric education. <u>Journal of Nervous
    and Mental Disease</u>, 154, 153-156, 1972.
Cleghorn, J. and Levin, S. Training family therapists by setting
    learning objectives. <u>American Journal of Orthopsychiatry</u>,
    43, 439-446, 1973.
Cohen, R. L. and Henderson, P. B. Experiences in the alteration
    of sequence in child psychiatry training. <u>Journal of American
    Academy of Child Psychiatry</u>, 12, 441-460, 1973.
Constantine, L. L. Designed experience: A multiple, goal-directed
    training program in family therapy. <u>Family Process</u>, 15,
    373-387, 1976.
Ehrlich, F. M. Family therapy and training in child psychiatry.
    <u>Journal of American Academy of Child Psychiatry</u>, 12, 461-472
    1973.
Flomenhaft, K. and Carter, R. E. Family therapy training: Program
    and outcome. <u>Family Process</u>, 16, 211-218, 1977.
Garza-Guerrero, A. C. Culture shock: Its mourning and the
    vicissitudes of identity. <u>Journal of American Psychoanalytic
    Association</u>, 22, 208-429, 1974.
Klagsbrun, S. C. In search of an identity. <u>Archives of General
    Psychiatry</u>, 16, 286-289, 1967.
Leon, R. L. The generation gap--Adult and child psychiatry.
    <u>Psychiatric Opinion</u>, 15, 37-39, 1978.
Malone, C. A. Observations on the role of family therapy in child
    psychiatric training, <u>Journal of American Academy of Child
    Psychiatry</u>, 13, 437-458, 1974.
McDermott, J. F., Jr. and Char, W. F. The undeclared war between
    child and family therapy. <u>Journal of American Academy of
    Child Psychiatry</u>, 13, 422-436, 1974.
Myerstein, I. Family therapy training for paraprofessionals in
    a community mental health center. <u>Family Process</u>, 16,
    477-493, 1977.
Montalvo, B. Aspects of live supervision. <u>Family Process</u>, 12,
    343-359, 1973.

Sharaf, M. R. and Levinson, D. J. The quest for omnipotence in
    professional training. Psychiatry, 27:135-149, 1964.
Wheelis, A. The Quest for Identity. New York:Norton, 1958.

PRODUCTIONS

TRAINING ISSUES FACED BY BOTH PSYCHOANALYSIS AND FAMILY THERAPY:

DISCUSSION OF DR. GOTTLIEB'S PAPER

Richard N. Atkins, M.D.

Downstate Medical Center

Brooklyn, New York

When Dr. Flomenhaft asked me to discuss Dr. Gottlieb's paper, he must have anticipated my response. He must have guessed that giving this paper to me, a person trained at length in psychoanalysis, and a person, who, in his own professional identity, struggles most exclusively with psychoanalytic theory, would generate a few sparks of enthusiastic response. For I do have a deep and abiding respect for psychoanalysis and for the legacy of genius that Sigmund Freud and others gave to our field. I am not a family therapist. It is an understatement to say that what I do not know about family therapy or general systems theory would fill volumes. Hence, I am at a decided disadvantage when compared to Dr. Gottlieb, who is obviously familiar with many issues in dynamic theories and therapy--as indicated by his careful and thoughtful paper.

I thought for a while about discussing some of the more traditional issues which separate psychoanalysis and family therapy, particularly my reservations about the capacity of family therapy or general systems theory to foster the kind of true understanding which produces dynamic intrapsychic change in a patient's psychic being. However, I find it more pressing to talk about some of the training issues which this paper implicitly raises, issues which rather than separate psycho-analysis and family therapy, make them unfortunately all too similar.

Dr. Gottlieb begins, I think quite rightly, in suggesting that our job as educators is to help the burgeoning child psychiatrist derive a professional identity. Citing Allen Wheelis' (1966) incisive monograph on identity, Dr. Gottlieb

191

suggests that a professional identity, as any identity, is <u>a</u> <u>coherent sense of self, the clarity of which derives from the</u> <u>dependable linkage of one's actions with one's values</u>. Now that point, the linkage of one's actions with one's values, deserves some serious thought.

In our academic environments, value is attached, with some reasonable rationale, to the amount and quality of training experiences. Dr. Gottlieb, I'm sure, values his training and expertise in family therapy, just as I value my training and capacity in psychoanalysis. To a reasonable extent, we would, I think, define our professional identities as family therapist and psychoanalyst respectively. And at that point, we may be on the brink of a difficulty which I think has been handled in less than fully desirable ways by psychoanalysts and family therapists. The difficulty is this: Once we begin to increasingly objectify a professional identity, we begin, almost by definition, to reify it. This would be an undesirable marriage between values and actions. Ernst Schachtel, in his paper: "On Alienated Concepts of Identity" (1961) outlines the problem as follows:

> "By making some quality or circumstance, real or exaggerated or imagined, the focal point of a reified identity, I look upon myself as though I were a thing and the quality or circumstance were a fixed attribute of this thing or object. But the "I" that feels that I am this or that, in doing so, distances itself from the very same reified object attribute which it experiences as determining its identity. In feeling that I am such and such, I distinguish between the I and the presumably unalterable quality which, for all time, condemns me to have this identity. I do not feel that <u>I am doing</u> this or that or failing to do it, but there <u>is</u> a something in me or about me, and that this once and for all, <u>makes</u> me this or that, fixes my identity."

In a similar way, who we are as psychotherapists can become wedded in an unfortunate manner to what we read, to what we infer as a metapsychology, to identifications (wholesale or partial) with charismatic teachers or personal or supervising therapists, or to that body of information which so often gets labeled technique or theory. Not that technique, theory, metapsychology, and teachers aren't vital. Indeed, Dr. Gottlieb points out their importance to a trainee as part-identificatory way-stations toward the development of true identifications which foster individuation and autonomy as a <u>doer</u> of psychotherapy.

But such <u>part-identifications</u>, or <u>pseudoidentifications</u>, to use David Schecter's (1968) felicitous phrase, can lead our professional selves into a closely merged relationship with a reified system of theoretical and technical values, where the values begin to dictate something of our identities and our actions. In short, theory or technique become theology, and therapists, rather than becoming active participant-observers, become embedded to a "higher calling."

Let me offer an example. There is a reasonable body of practical lessons and experience which is called psychoanalytic technique. There is a body of knowledge called psychoanalytic theory, some of it soundly based in clinical and developmental experience, some of it based in elaborate mechanistic and phylo-genetic conjecture--I think partly because the oral tradition of psychoanalysis is that a therapist should never be caught needing to answer a clinical question with "I don't know." And, in the clinical setting, there is also the therapist and there is the patient. In that clinical setting, the therapist must put himself in an <u>allocentric</u> position, fully open to and equidistant from his theory, his technique, and his patient--but with his attention directed always at his patient--child or adult--and that patient's experience with living. This is what I think Freud had in mind when he wrote of "evenly hovering attention." I know that, insofar as a therapist keeps himself "tuned in" to his patient's experience and his own experience with his patient, that his theory and his technique will march right along with him. Neither will forsake him, nor does he need, except as we all have human needs, to hide <u>autocentrically</u> embedded behind his theory or technique for salvation. The temptation to revert to autocentric perceptions lies in our need to <u>understand</u> our patients' experiences often before these are fully elaborated, or worse yet, to prematurely explain these kinds of understandings to our patients. We do this, significantly, because we have such problems tolerating the anxiety of facing the unknown and uncertain as our patients reflect that aspect of their experience toward us. And we have anxious difficulty in containing our patients' anxieties as they struggle to relate awesome dynamisms of psychic existence to themselves and to us.

Lawrence Friedman (1978), from Cornell, recently analyzed a published fragment of an analysis done by D. W. Winnicott, a man revered by me and certainly a revered name in our field. Despite the formidable brilliance of the analysis, even Winnicott was not exempt from the reification problem. Winnicott's occasional consuming interest in the "holding environment" and, in this particular case, with castration anxiety as well--led him to formulate his interventions almost exclusively in terms of the patient's needing to be held, and being, or fearing being, castrated--even when the <u>depths</u> of the patient's experience was

clearly going in alternative directions. Too much reliance
seems to have been placed on this therapist's picking up incomplete
cues from his patient which became compatible with an overvalued
mystical patient of the therapist's fantasy. And pieces of the
analysis became the effort to wed the fantasied patient with
one in actuality.

        Now, having said all of this, what has it to do with
training? Well, for better or for worse, and, I've suggested,
it's not always for the better, analysts love to explain clinical
phenomena. The legacy of theory and the metapsychology lure us
into all kinds of explanations, some of them indeed rather
mysteriously magical—especially if theory and metapsychology
become quasi-religious. And, if we teachers in the field are
liable to the anxiety of the unknown which the patient conjures
up for us, are our trainees exempt from similar difficulties?
Dr. Gottlieb points out two or three examples of how trainees
manage the anxiety of "not knowing" in the early part of his
paper. Certainly psychoanalytic theory and metapsychology
become, for many trainees, a safe haven for explanations. No
wonder it's so attractive. And for the analysts so imbued with
an autocentric philosophy, disciples are divine. No wonder, as
Dr. Gottlieb alludes, residents and fellows often enter into
the late arriving family therapy matrix with a relieving belief
system already sewn up.

        Now I turn to family therapy. Dr. Gottlieb suggests that
one way of combating the exclusive domain of psychoanalysis is to
introduce family therapy early in training programs--during the
summer when we know so many East Coast analysts, me among them,
have already caravaned to Cape Cod, and are out of the picture.
Well where psychoanalytic identity could suffer from a reification
of theory and metapsychology, I feel, empirically, that family
therapy suffers from a reification in technique--and this is how
it fights in a war which in itself might best be disbanded.
Family therapy has an occasionally overvalued marriage to its
tools, such as its one-way mirror treatment rooms, its two-way
intercoms, telephones, multiple-track tape recorders so that one
can hear supervisory comments overriding patient comments, its
multiple therapists, quasi-legal contracts, its sculpting, its
provocative seating arrangements where therapists, supervisors,
and patients move frequently into and out of the treatment
setting and change roles and seating arrangements with great
frequency. This kind of technical business can definitely provide
trainees with a very exciting alternative to psychoanalytic
therapy. It is not that I always anticipate reification, but
these techniques seem so highly invested in process and procedure
that I think this kind of reification, likewise in its artifi-
ciality, interferes with the true business of making sense out

of a patient's experiences with life. Shouldn't we begin to
worry that, on both fronts of this implicit "war" between reified
psychoanalysis and reified family therapy, we as educators are
disavowing our true professional identities? Certainly I
worry about giving our students any kind of overvalued "it" with
which to identify that can become the object of greater interest
than the "who" residing within them and their patients.

REFERENCES

Friedman, L. Presentation to the William Alanson White Psycho-
      analytic Society, New York, 1978.
Schecter, D. E. Identification and individuation Journal of the
      American Psychoanalytic Association, 1968, 16:48-80.
Schachtel, E. On alienated concepts of identity. American
      Journal of Psychoanalysis, 1961, 21:120 - 127.
Wheelis, A. The Quest for Identity. New York:Norton, 1966.

IS THE TASK OF INTEGRATING RESERVED FOR THE TRAINEE? GENERAL

DISCUSSION

DR. CHRIST

Thank you Dr. Atkins. That was a nice pulling together of a number of very important points which hopefully we will pursue.

DR. COMBRINCK-GRAHAM

I once had an anatomy professor who made this disclaimer of himself as a teacher in his anatomy course. Faced with first year medical students who were young adults, he said, "You cannot teach them anything. You can just provide a setting for them to learn in and they gotta do the learning themselves." I think that Dr. Atkins' paper refers to something that has been an underlying theme here, which is a certain arrogance of the psychiatric profession. I believe my anatomy professor was speaking about the mistaken arrogance of teachers. For physicians, this arrogance is, I guess, encouraged by the patients. But it puts the psychiatrist in the position of knowing more about the patients than the patients know about themselves, of being able to formulate the patient's problems better than the patient, of being able to instruct parents how to manage their children better than they do, and to tell them things about their children that they do not know. I think that this is a mistake which we all make at one time or another. I want to emphasize that one of the reasons I do family therapy is because I see the family as the child's major resource in his young life, and it is my intention to make that resource come to life in the best way it can. And I hope as I grow more mature to more successfully avoid instructing the family about how to do that.

AUDIENCE MEMBER

I am a second year fellow at the Philadelphia Guidance Clinic and I trained at Downstate Medical Center. I would just like to share with you a perspective from a child fellow who has been exposed to both an analytic orientation as a resident and now a family therapy orientation as a child fellow.

197

I think that some of the things that Drs. Gottlieb and Atkins touched upon are quite accurate, but they are from a different perspective, and the person who has to integrate it on the front lines is a person who is going through the process of learning a certain identity. Now Dr. Lee Combrinck-Graham spoke earlier about the depression that the first year fellows go through. Well I do not look at it so much that way, but as more of a developmental crisis that they go through. I would like to share with you briefly my first year experiences:

In the morning, at 9:00 A.M., I was exposed to a diagnostic seminar conducted by an analytically oriented teacher where I had to put together a family and analytic perspective. At 10:00 A.M., I would have a child come in with the mother where I would want my live supervisor to focus upon a developmental analysis of the child, who had a congenital heart defect, and, in addition to that, appeared retarded with autistic features. The supervisor, however, wanted me to focus more upon the diadic relationship of the husband and the wife, although the husband was not present. At noon, I would have an emergency where I had to do a psychiatric evaluation of a psychotic child from a psychiatric perspective, taking off my hat as a family therapist. Then at 2:00 o'clock, I would become a social worker when I am at a team meeting with other people about getting a kid into school, trying to coordinate child-life counselors, psycho-ed specialists, a psychologist and a whole group of others along with people from the public school system. At 3:00 o'clock, I would see an anorectic patient, and treat her individually to separate her from her family. At 4:00 o'clock, I could become a psychiatrist again from a psycho-pharmacological point of view in medication clinic, and then a student again in the medication clinic seminar. Then at 6:00 o'clock, I might be called to do a consultation at Children's Hospital where you become a physician when you see a psychotic girl who has a chronic brain syndrome. You detect organicity, and it turns out that she has lupus psychosis.

Within a period of ten hours, I have functioned as a psychiatrist, social worker, systems family therapist, and psycho-pharmacologist. Clearly, this produces a certain strain. Simultaneously, I have to learn how to begin to integrate all of this as I switch from role to role to role.

Supervisors have to learn to be sensitive to some of this switching phenomenon. I also would like to have the training directors think about that as well as the supervisors when they begin to consider the product that they are working on. Thank you.

DR. CHRIST

A very nice sequence of experiences! You left out a couple
of others. You might have to also do remedial education with
brain damaged youngsters, during which you have to worry about
what part of the brain you are tampering with. You point out
accurately that child psychiatry is still a mostly unintegrated
series of perspectives and techniques that our diverse patient
population forces us to be cognizant of. The single $E=MC^2$
formulation that draws together these diversities is not yet
available in our field. In the meantime, our biggest problem is
not eclecticism, but amateurish eclecticism. You point out
nicely the confusion that is inherent in the multiple approaches
you must use in a single day. I sense from your comments that
your lack of expertise in each of the areas, clearly to be
expected during one's training, adds to your discomfort. It is
a discomfort I respect, because it will goad you to develop
competent eclecticism!

AUDIENCE MEMBER

Welcome to child psychiatry for the resident who had all
those experiences. And I say this with empathy, warmth, and
generosity. Mind you, I do not say this in terms, "You know we
went through it, you have to go through it too." But maybe it
represents some distance that occurs.

The seasoned veteran is one who is mustered by the officers
and peppered up by the enemy. Perhaps the supervisor can become
too comfortable in his office. Maybe, every once in a while, the
supervisor has to break out of that frame and come with you as
a trainee for a day to see how anxious you get as you deal with
these varied clinical responsibilities. What is predominant in
your thinking? What do you think is your first priority? It
would be good if the supervisor were there to answer some of the
questions you have about taking a family approach when you have
to deal immediately with the retarded child, or the psychotic
child, or the team conference to decide the child's school
program.

That might help to bring you a little closer together with
the supervisor. I think you need more of that. You also need
some free time to be with the supervisor where you do not talk
about anything related to your work. Not enough of that is done
either. We do not have enough time to play with each other, as
well as with ideas about children and families. Maybe we have to
do something about the family of supervisors and students that
we do not recognize.

<u>DR. CHRIST</u>

I think we are beginning to touch on one of the terribly
difficult problems in training whether we as teachers feel
we can do the integrating, whether full integration is possible,
or whether integration is even good or not. Unfortunately the
trainee ends up having to do some of this. Our challenge as
educators is to find a way by which we can facilitate that
process for the trainee.

ISSUES POSED BY THE SYMPOSIUM: A DIALOGUE

The symposium concludes with a discussion by the presenters
and members of the audience. This is their first real opportunity
to dialogue with each other and pursue in depth the ideas,
issues, and dilemmas which have developed during these two days.

DR. CHRIST

Let us begin by questions from the audience.

AUDIENCE MEMBER

As a child fellow, I find in this symposium that some
people seem to see family therapy as a treatment modality;
others view family therapy as a way of thinking about problems.
Could the panel members further clarify this?

DR. COMBRINCK-GRAHAM

I believe that the theory of thinking about a person in
the context of his family or in the context where he lives is a
different theory from thinking about the person responding to
whatever is going on inside of him. There are major differences.
If the person responds to his context or develops or grows in a
context are a primary way that you think about people and their
dysfunctions, then the practice that is derived is automatically
going to involve major consideration of the family. It does not
necessarily mean that you do not do individual treatment. Our
family therapy trainees do a lot of individual treatment at the
Philadelphia Child Guidance Clinic but we also have a very
consistent focus on the ecology of the people that we treat. This
is not the same language as the language of psychoanalysis and
I think we have made a choice. You cannot speak two languages
at the same time. We teach a language of thinking about and
treating children which has to do with children and their
context.

DR. BROWN

     I would also like to consider the question but with a
slightly different emphasis. There is what might be called
cheap eclecticism and there is sophisticated eclecticism. Most
of us in the room are devoted to what I believe is a sophisticated
eclecticism. Therefore, it is not a question of a little piece
of family therapy and than a little piece of this and a little
piece of that, but rather a comprehensive understanding of the
needs of the patient, and within that comprehensive understanding,
the introduction of what is clinically pertinent.

     A case comes to mind which illustrates the point. A very
experienced psychoanalytically trained psychotherapist asked me
if I would see the Jones family. The mother was currently a
patient of her's. In the family were three children: one girl
was 12, one girl 10, and a little boy of about five whom I
thought of as the "little shitter." He was forever soiling his
pants and he was the target of the greatest overt distress in the
family--and a serious embarrassment to his two older sisters.
But the two sisters also had their problems. Now the individual
therapist of the mother felt that her effectiveness had begun to
reach a plateau in her psychodynamic therapy with the mother,
because the pervasive confusion in the family together with the
confusion within this woman in her role as mother was pre-
empting the analytic therapy that my colleague was trying to
carry out with her.

     When I saw the entire family, including, of course, both
parents and the three kids, it felt like a tornado of activity
hit my office. Half-way through the first session, I said to
the kids (not to the parents) "...you know, you are like an
upside down family." This immediately stopped the tornado and
the verbal confusion. The two older kids wanted to know what did
I mean and why did I say "we are an upside down family?" I
explained that the family is all upside down because the kids are
controlling the parents. I said, "...everything your parents
say, you ride right over and you pay no attention...so it's like
there are no parents--like you children are the parents...."

     At each subsequent family meeting, one or another of the
kids wanted to know, "Do you still think they were an upside
down family?" In due course, they stopped being an upside down
family. They settled down with much more internal regulation and
control. The little brother no longer shit in his pants on the
school bus and everywhere else. The mother continued in her
individual dynamic analytic therapy with much greater effect.
The father was already in group therapy and claimed he was getting
much more out of it after we began the family meetings. This

is an illustration of what I would call sophisticated eclecticism.
In this instance family thinking re: case management began not
from me, but from the individual analytic therapist.

DR. GOTTLIEB

You are trying to distinguish family therapy as a way of
thinking or family therapy as a way of doing therapy? It may
be important to make that distinction, but I do not see the boundary
as so clear maybe as you do. What I try to say is that they are
almost inseparable. If we teach people to do effective therapy
with children, thinking of them in context, the trainees will
achieve that kind of familial developmental orientation. They
may evolve their own model, like Dr. Brown's model, or perhaps
some other model which is more felicitous to them. But the
therapy experientially will provoke the thought processes. On
the other hand, you can go at it in quite the other way. If
you like cerebration or cognition, you start with a theory
with a certain developmental perspective, and by looking at these
particular task cycle issues, you then derive certain implications
for your practice and then you try those out. So at any one
time, if you are going to make a split between theory and
practice, one is going to be a little ahead of the other or a
little behind the other. But they really are very closely
linked and I think it is a mistake to try to make them too
separate.

DR. FLOMENHAFT

We as teachers have to be clear when we talk about family
theory and therapy and individual theory and treatment to
explicate the assumptions and the concepts associated with these
two discrete theories of thinking about people and problems.
Someone may say they are doing family therapy by seeing the whole
family, but view the family as a collection of individuals
rather than as an interactive, systemic unit. There is a set
of assumptions associated with each theory which evolves into
a differentiated practice model.

AUDIENCE MEMBER

I would like to say something about how to become a
sophisticated eclectic. There are certain things that are
conducive to becoming a good therapist, and one of the things is
learning one theory and technique well, regardless whether it
is an analytic model or it is a structural family therapy model.
One of the reasons I decided to go to the Philadelphia Child
Guidance Clinic is because I came from an eclectic institution.
I had no orientation and I realized that being a person with a

tendency to look at the broader perspective, I needed to focus
on one thing.

The second thing is that when I talk about family therapy,
I am really talking about systems. Regardless of whether I am
dealing with an individual alone who can be a system unto
himself, or a family within a larger system, it is all a systems
perspective. So I think psychoanalysis relevant to an individual
is dealing with a system of a different order, some would call
it a sub-system. Language is not too important to me. I have
seen family therapists who feel that it is against the law to
deal with individuals and I have seen family therapists who get
uncomfortable when they have to deal with the macro system
involving the school.

One of the things I learnt from my mentor in history of
medicine was that the differences concerning theory and technique
are usually not as great as simply just resting upon having a
different perspective. This was summed up in what my mentor
had told me about a chancellor of a large medical center who
had two lawyers. He needed a "yes" lawyer and a "no" lawyer. If
he wanted a negative opinion he gave it to his "no" lawyer; if
he wanted an affirmative position, he gave it to his "yes"
lawyer. And that is how I view this whole fight between analysts
and systems therapists.

AUDIENCE MEMBER

Most of the comments made so far have side stepped the
issue completely. The chancellor may have had two lawyers,but
he chose one; and he, apparently, did not say how he went about
choosing which one. In fact it did not really matter whether
the lawyers were there or not; it was his choice yes or no. I
think that a distinction between theory and technique is a clear
one and if we are going to talk about technique there is no
argument. There is no disagreement because we will just have
different opinions about which technique applies when and where.
What we have not talked much about is how do we go about making
this kind of decision? For example, I think Dr. Brown said
that there are some cases which are family cases and there are
some cases which are individual cases, but nothing was said about
how do you make the choice between the two. Thus far in the
symposium, the two approaches or the theories remain as noted
by Jay Hayley "incompatible." There has been no area of agreement.
One theory in fact contradicts the other and that issue has not
been addressed as far as I have seen. If one is true, then the
other is not.

DR. BROWN

I made an effort in that direction but I do not assume that
it really answers your point. I was hoping to show how my
emphasis on developmental sequence and its inevitability leads
me to decisions about which modality to use at a given time.
Developmental change occurs within a context and that context
itself is always changing. This must be constantly kept in
mind by the therapist. The job of the therapist, then, is to
discern where the resistance to change in that context is operating,
and with what degree of energy and impact. This is just another
way of talking about a family system. Now if the resistance to
change in the context or the system is principally a function of
individual psychopathology in a particular member of the family
even though peaking, so to say, at this particular time in the
family's developmental cycle, the most useful intervention might
be individual psychodynamic therapy for that person and not
clinical effort with the family as a whole, even if he or she is
having great current impact in that family field and is effectively
creating a resistance to normal developmental change in the system.
For example, I observed in the Jones family, a recurring nonpsy-
chotic depressive state in the father. His depressions had
enormous impact upon the marriage, upon the interactions between
the children, upon his role as a father and upon the family
system's development. Nevertheless, after having closely surveyed
this family field through the use of family interviews, I might
decide to say to the family "Look, there are lots of problems
I see...." I would describe some of them.   But then I would
say: "...I think you need to understand that the depression in
you, Mr. Jones, is affecting everyone at this time in the life of
your family and I think this is what you need help for to begin
with." Implicit in this--and I might state it explicitly--is
that for the family as a whole to make progress, father's
depression needs to be dealt with but other's problems will also
require attention a little later. Here is a choice toward
individual therapy arriving out of a clinical survey of that
family field. I use the concept of resistance to developmental
change as a background and guideline for my thinking and from
there, define what is most useful right now.

DR. CHRIST

How many dimensions do we really need if we call ourselves
complete psychiatrists? For example, I am thinking of a young
man who has total memory loss secondary to brain damage. This
happened when he was eight; he is now about 14. The family is
affected; the youngster is affected; the school situation is
affected; and I am affected. I am affected because I have to
try to figure out how to do treatment with somebody who has no
memory. In order to help this young man, I have had to do a lot

of reading about the brain, its parts, its operation and a lot
of stuff having to do with cognition. In order to be a holistic
psychiatrist, I am not sure yet how many dimensions are necessary.
I know that two, the psychoanalytic and the family perspectives,
are not enough.

DR. EHRLICH

I think this question that you ask gets to the heart of the
matter. Is there a real fundamental theoretical difference? Are
there really two schools of thinking, two ways of looking at
this data which are incompatible and even contradictory? I
myself do not think so. I think, in fact, that practice is
often more incompatible than theory. I am impressed that often
when you get a detailed report of the way that someone works, it
is not as different from what you do as you think it is when you
hear about his or her theory. The reason that the two theories
are not incompatible, the psychoanalytic and the transactional
theory, is that there is an artificial separation. When one sees
a patient in individual therapy or in analysis and you achieve an
affective contact with that other individual, you really are then,
totally there in touch with your patient and feel that something
is happening. For that moment, the rest of the world is in
suspension. You have no awareness, contact or interest in anything
else. It is as if for that moment only the two of you existed in
the universe. Now, clearly, you both know that that is not so,
but at that intense moment of absorption, it is as if the rest
of the world did not exist. Similarly, in a family interview,
where there is that moment of affective content, everybody in the
room is to some extent experiencing something simultaneously,
that intense hushed moment which Dr. Brown talked about when he
said, "the upside down family." You can almost feel it, like a
mystical feeling and the atmosphere changes. At that moment,
it is as if no one existed as a separate individual; all that
exists is the interaction on what is happening among everybody.
Now everyone knows that somewhere if you stop and think about it,
everyone is an individual but no one feels like an individual. It
is being able to move from the artificial assumption that one
exists alone in the universe and nothing else exists, to moving
to the artificial assumption that what exists is only the interaction but knowing always that the other is there. That makes
the two theories compatible.

DR. GOTTLIEB

Having surveyed this family field, a therapist can make a
choice of where to address the impediments, the processes of major
resistances to change and then he goes towards them. That
survey of the family field is not a public opinion survey;

it is not even a family opinion poll and it is not a survey, I
hope, of colleagues' therapeutic prejudices. The survey occurs
because the surveyor, the one who is doing the evaluation of this
family field, has the skills to obtain the reference points that
you need to get to do a survey. I, clearly, believe that it is
important that the surveyor knows he is an active and an
intrinsic part of that field. He has become a part of the field
under observation. He tests out certain notions about where an
intervention is likely to pay off or not, by making minor interventions as he goes. And that then gives him new feedback data
about what the terrain is like in the family field. The problem
with looking at the field from some of the other perspectives
which have been alluded to is that the therapist might have a
notion they are somehow surveyors from afar without getting into
the field and being able to do the kind of survey of what is going
on in this family which then can result in making an effective
recommendation. Family members can be interviewed individually,
in dyads some of the time, and conjointly at times. That is not
at all the issue. The issue is how the therapist learns to
assimilate, accumulate and precipitate the exposure of those data
to his wise perspective. There are therapists who believe you
should not try any intervention until you have gathered an
enormous amount of diagnostic information. There are other
therapists who believe that as soon as you open the door, you
start intervening; you got a smell and a sense from the way the
family is sitting, and the way the family is talking together,
and that this is a family that has a problem with X, Y, or Z.
And very rapidly, you then may begin to test out your hypothesis.
That is an active therapist intervening in a situation calculated
to obtain more data and information about what longer range
therapeutic interventions are likely to be successful.

AUDIENCE MEMBER

     I am a first year child fellow in the throes of soul searching
about which theories and family therapy I should follow. What
I would like to get from my training program is to have my
supervisors be clear about the theories that they are trying
to impart and then be allowed to pursue what I want to do as a
therapist later on.

DR. CHRIST

     Let me make sure I understand exactly what you are saying.
In other words, you would like from your supervisors a clear
sense of what the various theories are and what the various
theoretical positions are? You would like then the freedom to
be able to choose which one you want?

DR. COMBRINCK-GRAHAM

I am very concerned about the blurring of the distinctions that I personally have tried so hard to keep separate. I do not think that you can teach family therapy, good family therapy, with a good family theory, in a training program that is primarily wedded to individual psycho-dynamic theory. You cannot do it and it is unfair and confusing to the fellows. Our fellows at the Philadelphia Child Guidance Clinic went through something like this last year when one of the major teachers in our program had a primarily psychodynamic orientation. As a result, the trainees were excessively confused. At the level of education of a child psychiatry trainee, it is irresponsible not to have a primary point of view and expect the students to select the program for this.

Fellows come to the Child Guidance Clinic because they know what to expect; they will go to another program if they want to get another kind of emphasis. As educators, it is our responsibility to be clear about a perspective and to make it very clear in the prospectus that we send potential students, and then to be very clear in the way we proceed to teach it. My experience is that when one has both approaches to child psychiatry training in the same program, the fellows do not sufficiently adopt the paradigm of family thinking and family therapy to be really proficient. That is, of course, if you believe that family therapy is more than seeing the individuals together in a family group.

DR. BROWN

We have lost track of an important strand in making this differentiation. Formulated somewhat puristically, the keystone of analytic type one-to-one therapy is the transference. One hopes for the opportunity to work with the transference that evolves in the context of an individual patient meeting with an individual psychodynamic analytic therapist. This is the core of a traditional psychodynamic psychotherapy, one-to-one. The family systems orientation with its focus on interactions among several people is a very different frame of reference and the trainee faces a considerable degree of cognitive challenge and potential confusion in integrating these during early phases of the learning experience. If the supervisors are psychoanalytically immersed, they are likely to repeatedly ask a trainee, "What is happening in the transference?" This, after all, is a dominant theme of good dynamic therapy. In family therapy, the question of what is happening in the transference is almost never raised. If it is raised, it usually is immediately discussed in terms of how it is played out in the intrafamilial transactions, rather than between the therapist and any single family member.

On the other hand, I would like to emphasize that the concepts of counter-transference are absolutely essential for family therapy. If I supervise someone doing family therapy or if someone were supervising me, I would want questions to come up often about my counter-transference reactions to the various members of the family as well as to the family as a totality. The supervisors' question needs to be: "How are you experiencing the people in the family?" As a supervisor, I would not intend to be analyzing the trainee; I would only want to know if the trainee is in touch with his or her "counter-transference reactions."

A common transference theme that comes up in individual therapy is the idealization of the therapist. Ordinarily, in individual therapy, I might accept that idealization for many sessions unless it interferes with progress. If it does, I would make some interpretation early in the therapy. Either way, my aim would be to help the patient recognize firstly that he or she is idealizing me; and secondly that the need to do this has meaning for him based upon his particular history. What I am describing is a psychoanalytic type of response to the common phenomenon of transference idealization. In contrast to this, what is the focus in family therapy when someone in the family begins to idealize me? If the mother says, "Let's ask Dr. Brown what he thinks..." I might respond, "...look what's happening--you seem to erase what your husband said and you turn to me as if I know everything--but what's going on between the two of you?" The point is that what begins to sound like a transference involvement with me should, in family therapy, be deflected back into the family interaction.

DR. EHRLICH

One of our problems is of vocabulary and it gets quite important. Transference and counter-transference are words that really come from analysis and have very specific technical meanings. We tend to use them very loosely just as "acting out" has come to be common parlance now, and yet it has a very specific meaning initially; "acting up" might be better or "behaving badly." What goes on in a conjoint family meeting does not have the same quality of individual, regressive recreating of the infantile world which is the specific goal of the individual therapy or the analytic situation. What goes on in a family meeting is a very different business. And there are certainly distortions, idealizations and differences in the way the therapist may be perceived, but by using the word "transference," we too easily make identities out of things which are different. And to ask a trainee or ask ourselves, "My God, how do I feel when that happens in a family meeting?" is quite different from asking about counter-transference

issues which are not simply conscious, impulsive responses that
one is aware of in reaction to what is going on, but represent a
whole complex of regressive often unconscious responses in the
therapist.

AUDIENCE MEMBER

After eight years of trying to introduce family therapy in
three different settings, I am in a dilemma. Do I go in there
and very dramatically say this is the way it is going to be? If
you do not do it my way, I am going to leave; or I am going to
use every kind of method that I have to manipulate this into
the curriculum? Or should I, in a very gradual way, expose what
I am trying to do and enter people into discussions around it
all? I tried them both and, frankly, I have been frustrated with
both approaches. I am wondering if the panel might address this?
How does one introduce family therapy into a system?

DR. FLOMENHAFT

I remember Carl Whittaker telling me that he tried going at
it like gang busters in Atlanta and was run out of town. Then
he went up to Wisconsin and he took the soft sell. After eight
years, he felt he made some progress because he met an analyst in
the men's room who asked him to see a family.

DR. BROWN

I would like to push a point though. It is the soft sell
appropos what was said about Whittaker. At my institution, we
recently organized the adult outpatient clinic service delivery
system. First year residents are assigned to multidisciplinary
teams which include social workers, psychologists, doctoral
fellows. There are approximately eight on the team. At least
half are in training. An evaluation of a case can go up to six
sessions. Those in training have the option to use those six
sessions not only for the designated patient, but also for meeting
conjointly or independently with the spouse, family, mate, or
whatever. The team then reviews the evaluations and formulates a
consensus about case management. If on each team there is at
least one person who while not necessarily a family therapist, is
nevertheless receptive to and aware of the value of family interviewing, the ecology of the team becomes tilted, so to speak, in
the direction of including direct contact with families as a part
of basic clinical work. As it turns out, this "takes" with some
trainees and not with others. Who is supervising their work
outside of the teams affects this considerably--i.e. who their
models are. Withal, by the end of the first year of residency,
or of doctoral training, most of the trainees have been encouraged
at least a number of times to see a patient's family. Their

experience may not always be successful, but hopefully, at least for many, the resistance to and the anxiety about meeting with a family has been reduced. In the case of our residents, some become interested in child psychiatry training. This is one variation of the "soft sell."

DR. EHRLICH

I think this is a terribly important question. My answer on the simplest level is that you have to do it the way you have to do it. Each training program has to have some coherence. I do not think people have to drive each other out but they may, and unless you can do it in a way that is you and work with people in a way that is them then you do not have a training program. And, there are many different ways.

I am a patient man, and for me it has been a pleasure to bit by bit see some of the people I have trained now on staff who are using more family techniques. First year adult residents working in the local V.A. hospital are all expected to see the families of the adults who are admitted, and they have child psychiatrists as supervisors with a family orientation. So bit by bit, things change and that for me is a better way. I get uneasy about dramatic sudden change because I have put a lot of importance on what I have been through and what we have learnt slowly. Other people, I think, can come in and make change in the right situation with the right person which may be a better way to do it. I do not think there is an easy answer.

AUDIENCE MEMBER

I always get disturbed as a teacher that there are some people who feel they know the truth; and I always assumed that there were truths. At the end of our two year child psychiatry training program, I hope the graduate is given some basic tools. My concept of child psychiatry is that you train the child psychiatrist to look at the child in a variety of systems. From what I have heard thus far in this symposium, I am afraid that the child is viewed primarily in the system of the family or the system of his individual psyche. What is overlooked is that the child is in the system of his physiology, is in a system of his school, is in a system of his community which have not really been addressed. My orientation is to look at the child in a holistic way.

DR. COMBRINCK-GRAHAM

Now in response to the other contexts in which children grow and develop, I did allude to them in my paper. I have highlighted the family in terms of contextual theory merely because it is the

family that is the most portable and a most manageable sized interpersonal context in which we find children.

AUDIENCE MEMBER

Dr. Brown made some very interesting remarks about the
developmental state of trainees. I wonder if other members of
the panel would comment on this?

DR. COMBRINCK-GRAHAM

I felt that Dr. Brown's characterization of the trainees stage
of development was really very well articulated. Fellows come
to a training program to learn what we can teach them which is a
body of theory and some practice based on that theory. But what
he had talked about was a lack of experience, and training programs
really are not supposed to give people life experience, the kind
of life experience associated with the passing of time and or
maturation. After I read his paper, I began to think about those
of us who entered our training programs, not married and with no
children of our own. People would say, "How can you be a child
psychiatrist if you do not have any children of your own?" We
were all children once and not only that but we all know a lot of
children. Furthermore, we have been to the movies; we have seen
a lot of families; and we have read about a lot of families.
And we see them on the bus every day or on the streets on or in
the waiting rooms, and there are just a vast variety of experiences
that we do have that we could be possibly making more use of in
the training.

In order to get people in touch with the experiences that
they do have, I tried last year by assigning each one of my first
year fellows to a normal family from a pediatric practice in which
there was at least one pre-school child and one newborn baby. It
turned out that the fellows did not find time to make use of that
experience. Everybody agreed that it was a wonderful opportunity,
but nobody really had the time to make use of that experience.
Probably, it is the tincture of time that ripens our fellows.

AUDIENCE MEMBER

What we have done in our own training program is that within
the family therapy seminar we have created essentially another
family. In fact, we were not aware of it until the trainees
brought it to our attention. What we have is essentially an
even mix between faculty and trainees from varied mental health
disciplines. Members of the faculty became fathers, mothers,
grandmothers, and it has been very useful to see how some of our
trainees became children, elderly children ready to leave the
training and the younger children looking up to them and envying

them but at times very much in rivalry with them. It has been very useful at the end of each one of our sessions to look at the process. Each one of us has the opportunity to report on the process of that particular session so that it then also allows us to step back and see what it is that went on in the family as we were discussing actual family cases.

My question is on a different track. One of the things that I find to be a major blockage in integrating family therapy into psychiatry and mental health work is that it is not officially recognized in our diagnostic nomenclature. We can discuss all we learned about family structures and dynamics but in the end we have to call the patients according to DSM II and from what I understand DSM III is not going to help us any further. So it does become a lot of talk because when it comes down to what can be said to the person who is going to be paying or the person who is going to be viewing our record is a diagnosis that somehow is not relevant about what we may feel about the family structure.

AUDIENCE MEMBER

Given the state of mind of third party payers, even if we sent them a family diagnosis and our diagnostic nomenclature we probably would not get paid because they would not know what the hell that damm psychiatrist was talking about. I think that is an area where there is a possibility with DSM IV but we are not going to do it in DSM III although it has been talked about and discussed in the committee. With DSM IV there should be an access for a description of the structure of the family or family diagnosis. I would prefer a description of the structure of the family. I doubt seriously that the third party payers are going to pay us in the next 50 years for doing family diagnosis. We still have to hide that you are actually seeing this whole family and the child and I am not comfortable with that either. This is one place we seriously need as child psychiatry educators to have an impact.

Also, what is our responsibility in terms of the child psychiatry boards to provide testing and demonstration of competency in family theory as well as family diagnosis as well as family therapy? And we have a real responsibility there because if we get it in there, it is in.

DR. CHRIST

From what I gather in the discussion thus far, there might be some interest in a triaxial classification in which family structure might be one of the components of a diagnostic formulation.

When you try to make a "complete" diagnosis, there might be up to six or seven diverse axes that need to be addressed.

DR. COMBRINCK-GRAHAM

I am a pragmatist and I know that to get paid for what you do, you have to have a diagnosis of a person. What our fellows usually do is put down three diagnoses. They put a DSM II diagnosis of the index child, a GAP diagnosis of the index child, and a diagnosis of a family using a one sentence description.

AUDIENCE MEMBER

Diagnosis in family therapy is still in the process of evolution. But we do have certain rubrics that we use which are descriptive and have certain dangers in them. For example, in psychosomatic families, one of the patterns that one often sees is enmeshment. Now you can have enmeshment in the family without a psychosomatic condition. But what happens is that because you expect this to be an enmeshed family, you begin to start looking a lot for enmeshment. We then have a tendency to start over-reading into a family something and we start deriving from it that the person has to have such and such so, therefore, they have such and such.

DR. CHRIST

I would like us to pursue further this issue of diagnostic system. I am trying to highlight what the ideal would be that each of us on the panel would go for. My prediction would be that Dr. Combrinck-Graham would opt for a unitary diagnosis which would be a family diagnosis. I would suspect Dr. Brown that your diagnostic ideal would be at least a two dimensional one and mine might be like a six dimensional one.

DR. COMBRINCK-GRAHAM

I would probably go for a unitary diagnosis that described the family. Nevertheless, one must keep in mind the previously mentioned dangers of a committee approved system and diagnostic vocabulary. Above all, I am very comfortable with the one sentence description of the way the family functions, especially if it avoids jargon like "enmeshment" or "rigid" or "over involved" that really may not have a great deal of meaning outside the walls of my institution, but is really an objective description of the way the family functions around the problem being presented.

<u>DR. CHRIST</u>

    I would like to thank all of you for your participation in
this conference. We have spoken about the teaching of Family
Therapy, and about the content of the teaching. We have heard
about various experiences in the introduction of Family Therapy,
and reached unanimity that the introduction should be gradual.
We have spoken at length about the integration of developmental,
psychoanalytic, and family concepts. All but one presenter
contributed to the question of how to conceptualize this integration. One presenter feels that only family concepts should be
taught, or, to state it more accurately, that there is place in
our various training centers for at least one that uses family
concepts as the exclusive orienting framework. We heard a
great deal that reflects the profound thinking and re-thinking
towards a further development of family theory. What particularly
impressed me was that the theorizing is no longer confined to the
parameters of the processes of family interaction, but, perhaps
because of the psychoanalytic orientation and/or training of most
of the participants, now includes developmental and metapsychological considerations.

    Finally, we spoke not only about what to teach, but how to
teach. I was impressed that there was great underlying agreement,
and that variations reflect more the availability of training
staff, of trainee time, and of administrative backing that results
in the financing of such teaching tools as one-way mirrors and
videotapes. Here, the tenor was more one of wanting to try an
innovative idea, wishing one had the trainee time to implement
ideas. The complement of didactic seminars with supervision,
always including some live, one-way mirror, or videotape supervision, is ubiquitous. Yesteryear's "dangers" of confidentiality,
of pure family OR individual therapy, now seem dead issues. Rather,
the preoccupation is when to use which modality with the same
family.

    As a beginning resident, I remember vividly Don Jackson and
Gregory Bateson describing their developing ideas about schizo-
phrenogenic mothers, the double bind theory, and the cybernetic
model. There has been a major increment in the sophistication
of family thinking since that time, as evidenced by these presentations.

    There are still many challenges left. Of particular concern
to us at Downstate Medical Center-Kings County Hospital, is the
place of family thinking and family therapy with the single parent
family, the minority member family, the multiproblem poverty or
welfare family, the young teenage mother-infant with, or as is
so often the case, without father, etc. Many of us who are not
identified as family therapists see the absolute necessity of

this modality in our treatment armamentaria, and want our trainees
to learn it. We also see the dire need for techniques applicable
to our multiproblem severely disorganized families. Perhaps
this can be the focus of our next symposium.

CONTRIBUTORS

Richard N. Atkins, M.D.   Clinical Assistant Professor
Director of Training
Division of Child & Adolescent
    Psychiatry
Downstate Medical Center-Kings
    County Hospital
Brooklyn, New York

Saul L. Brown, M.D.   Director, Department of Psychiatry
Cedars-Sinai Medical Center
Los Angeles, California

Richard Chasin, M.D.   Assistant Clinical Professor of
    Psychiatry
Boston University School of Medicine
Boston, Massachusetts

Adolph E. Christ, M.D.   Associate Professor
Director, Division of Child and
    Adolescent Psychiatry
Downstate Medical Center-Kings
    County Hospital
Brooklyn, New York

Lee Combrinck-Graham, M.D.   Assistant Clinical Professor
Director, Child Psychiatry Training
Philadelphia Child Guidance Clinic
Philadelphia, Pennsylvania

Frederick M. Ehrlich, M.D.   Associate Clinical Professor of
    Psychiatry
Tufts University School of Medicine
Boston, Massachusetts

Kalman Flomenhaft, Ph.D.   Clinical Associate Professor
                                  Director of Family Therapy
                                  Division of Child & Adolescent
                                      Psychiatry
                                  Downstate Medical Center-Kings
                                      County Hospital
                                  Brooklyn, New York

Wells Goodrich, M.D.   Director of Child and Adolescent
                                      Research
                                  Chestnut Lodge
                                  Rockville, Maryland

Fred Gottlieb, M.D.   Associate Professor of Psychiatry
                                  University of California Los Angeles
                                  Department of Psychiatry
                                  School of Medicine
                                  The Center for the Health Sciences
                                  Los Angeles, California

Henry Grunebaum, M.D.   Director, Group and Family Psycho-
                                      therapy Training
                                  Department of Psychiatry
                                  Cambridge Hospital
                                  Cambridge, Massachusetts

Donald G. Langsley, M.D.   Professor and Chairman
                                  Department of Psychiatry
                                  University of Cincinnati Medical
                                      Center
                                  Cincinnati, Ohio

Charles A. Malone, M.D.   Professor and Director
                                  Division of Child Psychiatry
                                  Case Western Reserve University
                                  Cleveland, Ohio

INDEX

219